"The Good Life is the new definition of holistic health—it's a book that will help change lives."

~ Deepak Chopra, author of *Jesus: A Story of Enlightenment*

"A book on health and well-being in a class of its own. Two thousand years ago, Epictetus, a Greek philosopher, introduced the notion that professional human beings could become skilled in the fine art of living. Twenty centuries later, Jesse Dylan and fifteen visionaries expand the concept in a mind-shifting narrative sparkling with gemlike insights. The breadth, depth and clarity of the ideas will leave the reader with a heightened awareness of human possibilities. Readers may also find themselves struck by an irresistible impulse to share their newfound wisdom with friends and family."

~ Carole Carson, author of *From Fat to Fit*

"Jesse Dylan has attracted the most amazing, powerful and influential leaders in the categories that matter most. It's brilliant—people will love this book!"

~ Leeza Gibbons, television and radio host

"In The Good Life, Jesse Dylan has gathered a perfect blend of viewpoints and guidelines for healthy living, from some of the most brilliant minds of our time. If you are searching for ideas to expand your consciousness in the areas of health, wealth and happiness, this book is a must read!"

~ Dannion and Kathryn Brinkley, authors of *Secrets of the Light: Lessons from Heaven*

"*The wisdom and practices in this book will usher you into a holistic way of life that supports your purpose on the planet—to flourish and glow as you deliver your talents, gifts and skills for the benefit of all beings.*"

~ Dr. Rev Michael Bernard Beckwith, author of *Spiritual Liberation: Fulfilling Your Soul's Potential*

"*A spiritual treasure trove of health and wellness insights from some of the most incredible thinkers on our planet*—The Good Life shines a light for those who want to truly attain health and happiness."

~ James O. Hill, Professor of Pediatrics, University of Colorado, Co-Founder of America on the Move and author of *The Step Diet Book*

"*The inspired thoughts and insights in* The Good Life *will help people create their dreams and live the abundant life they are meant to enjoy.*"

~ Dr. John Demartini, author of *The Riches Within*

"The Good Life with Jesse Dylan *is a powerful and in-depth integration of wisdom from outstanding visionaries and holistic thinkers of this era, covering the full spectrum of body, mind, and spiritual information and inspiration. It is a wonderful synergy that will support and encourage many into living the Good Life.*"

~ Gabriel Cousens, M.D., M.D.(H), Diplomat in Ayurveda, D.D., Rabbi, author of *There is a Cure for Diabetes* and the Director of the Tree of Life Rejuvenation Center

THE
GOOD LIFE

with

JESSE DYLAN

Redefining Your Health with
the Greatest Visionaries of Our Time

THE
GOOD LIFE
with
JESSE DYLAN

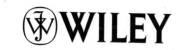

John Wiley & Sons Canada Ltd.

Library and Archives Canada Cataloguing in Publication Data
Dylan, Jesse
 The good life with Jesse Dylan : redefining your health with the greatest visionaries of our time / Jesse Dylan.

ISBN 978-0-470-15694-0

 1. Holistic medicine. 2. Health. 3. Mind and body. I. Title.
R733.D965 2009   613   C2008-907642-7

Production Credits
Cover design: Wendy Mount
Cover photo: Kevin Clark
Interior text design and typesetting: Adrian So
Printer: Tri-Graphic Printing, Ltd.

Editorial Credits
Editor: Leah Fairbank
Project Coordinator: Lindsay Humphreys

John Wiley & Sons Canada, Ltd.
6045 Freemont Blvd.
Mississauga, Ontario
L5R 4J3

Printed in Canada

1 2 3 4 5 TRI 13 12 11 10 09

To the love of my life—Jilli.
To my sons, Justin, Joshua and Joel.

Follow your dreams!

CONTENTS

SECTION 2: HEALTH OF BODY

SECTION 3: HEALTH OF SPIRIT

ACKNOWLEDGMENTS

This book has been a labor of love for me, as it fulfils my long-time desire to see the message of *The Good Life* enter important new avenues of expression. In its writing, I have counted on the help of a number of good friends and associates, and to them I want to extend my sincere gratitude. They have formed an incredible team; a small peaceful army of people who have helped or contributed at different stages. Therefore my thanks go out:

To the very special 15 guests of *The Good Life* show who agreed to appear in this book and who contributed to its completion, and to the many hundreds of others who have so graciously contributed their time and energy to the program over the years.

To the world's greatest executive producers, Sam and Robin Mednick, and to my writing partner and friend, Jim Grove (a "peaceful warrior" in his own right).

To Leah Fairbank and the fantastic "Team Wiley."

To the amazing Dea Shandera and the "The Visioneering Group."

To my mother, for her bravery and courage.

And most of all, to the listeners and now readers who have supported the flow of this information for all these years—your enthusiasm gives life to this work.

INTRODUCTION

We live at a time when new advances in our knowledge of human health and wellness are appearing at a staggering speed. Whether we look at medical science, exercise and fitness, diet and nutrition, psychology and mind, or spirituality, we find fresh information and insights emerging all the time that illuminate what it means to be human and truly healthy in all the dimensions of our being. The question for many of us in the face of all this information is: Where do we start? And how can we combine various health practices relating to body, mind, and spirit into one practical plan for our daily personal wellness?

In the 10 years that I have been hosting *The Good Life* radio program, my goal has been to provide listeners with the best available information in this growing field of holistic health. I have interviewed some of today's most prominent researchers, writers, and speakers in the medical, wellness, self-help, and spiritual fields in the process, in an effort to blend the very best in health, lifestyle, vital living, and transformational content for reaching our highest human potential. Why? Because we know that true health is about more than just a good diet, having a strong physique, and avoiding serious illness. Humans have a complex array of needs related to all three dimensions of who we are—mind, body, and spirit—and *The Good Life* has consistently addressed all three of those areas.

You could say that my guests on *The Good Life* form the nexus of the new paradigm of health consciousness. They reflect the movement toward holistic health that has been steadily reshaping our culture in recent decades, and is especially gaining momentum at the start of the twenty-first century. You have seen signs of it everywhere, particularly in new attitudes and openness toward progressive health and lifestyle practices that would have been greeted with derision by our mainstream culture only a couple of decades ago. Examples include the large numbers of people who are starting to explore alternative and Eastern exercises such as yoga and tai chi, others switching to vegetarian and vegan diets, and others finding new definitions of personal spirituality through global integrative approaches to faith. Unprecedented numbers of people are now adopting these and many other diverse practices as they seek a more comprehensive sense of wellness.

They have realized that a truly holistic definition must account for the three cardinal elements of health. To have strong and healthy bodies, we also need to have healthy minds. A healthy mind must be supported by a joyful, fulfilling spiritual life, and a healthy spiritual life can in turn influence our physical well-being. In short, all of these components combine to make individuals healthy as a whole. At the same time, there is also a greater expectation that individuals who are whole in body, mind, and spirit are essential in nurturing the health of our communities at large, and ultimately the well-being of the global community itself.

Most of us buy diet and fitness books in the hope that a healthier body will give us the energy and enthusiasm we seem to lack. When we see no change in our energy, we buy inspirational books about the secret to happiness or finding meaning in our lives, and we focus on trying to apply those lessons in isolation from an exercise program or good diet. Then we read about building better marriages, or generating material wealth, or finding our purpose in life, and we don't see how they relate to each other. And each time we pick up a new title, the previous books tend to recede from our memory as we focus our attention on the health topic at hand. Our fragmented picture of wellness makes no improvement; we glimpse things in narrow, disconnected fragments, and we get inconsistent results to match.

If we can integrate these different elements, we start to experience balanced, incremental growth in all aspects of our health simultaneously. This type of integration is taking place in virtually every field of learning, so it's not a trend limited to health. In disciplines such as psychology, history, technology, and economics, experts have become more vocal about the need to tear down the walls between their fields. It is increasingly recognized that our traditional segregated approach—focusing on one discipline in isolation from the rest—most often provides only a small window of useful insight into an issue. If we attempt to rely on these snippets of insight, we lose the broader perspective of a complete, interwoven understanding.

But there is change afoot. As we've seen on *The Good Life* for these past 10 years, incorporating these practices holds a key to finding lasting health. We stop attacking isolated problems in our lives, and we accept that every lifestyle choice affects the whole. By making changes that respect the holistic nature of our experience, every aspect of our overall health improves.

The first step is to ensure our health of mind, as it is our mind that mediates our physical activity and helps to frame our spiritual life. In chapters 1 to 6, we will discover techniques and habits for clarifying our thinking, finding happiness, and living with confidence. Next, we will address the needs of our physical body, the vehicle that allows us to engage in all of our worldly activities, as well as our mental and spiritual pursuits. In chapters 7 through 10, we will learn the secrets to nurturing our bodies so they will be strong, resilient to illness, able to age with grace, and be robust enough to carry us through the experiences of life. Finally, we need to recognize that our spiritual life ultimately shapes the overall health of our entire being. In chapters 11 to 15, we will receive insights into nourishing our spiritual natures as we learn about spiritual guidance, life purpose, and the transformational power of compassion and forgiveness.

This book and *The Good Life* program have grown in part out of my own journey into wellness of body, mind, and soul. For starters, I didn't always enjoy the physical health that I have today. Some years ago I was 75 pounds heavier and in pretty poor shape. You might say I was oversubscribed to living "the good life" of another variety. At that time, someone who took an interest in my well-being suggested that I take up running, so I did. I got so excited about running that I ended up competing in several marathons, including the New York City Marathon twice. I had so much fun that I decided to tackle triathlons, and I went on to compete in about 50 triathlons, including three as a member of the Canadian national team at the World Championships, as well as the World Long-Distance Championships in Nice, France.

It was during the latter race that I had an epiphany: What if I could combine my experience in radio broadcasting with my new love of health and wellness? This was the first inspiration in a series that would lead me to create the health and lifestyle network called *The Good Life*, and ultimately to pursue a deeper exploration of my own emotional and spiritual life that would include "synchronistic" encounters with great teachers such as Bob Proctor of *The Secret*. In the years since I started *The Good Life*, I've polished some of the rough edges that once characterized me as something of a radio "shock jock." I've become friends with many of the renowned authors and sages whom I have interviewed, and integrated new ways of thinking and being in the process. A number of my program guests originally suggested that I should write a book featuring the very best of the information that has come forward from our conversations.

This book is the fruit of that seed.

It has been an incredible privilege to learn from some of the greatest thinkers in the world of health and human potential. If you're ready to take their insights and knowledge to heart, you'll find you're on a better footing for living a longer, healthier, and more vibrant life in mind, body, and spirit. May their insights inspire and lead you to a greater experience of vitality and purpose.

SECTION 1

In the health triumvirate of body, mind, and spirit, your mind is the mediator between your physical body and your spiritual life. In the ideal expression of its middle-management role, the mind provides a practical link between the abstract realm of your soul experience and the pragmatic world of your daily physical life. If you enjoy a calm, untroubled mind, you will make wise choices and adopt habits to ensure your physical wellness, and you will more easily relinquish mental control when you encounter elements of spiritual experience that typically fall outside your conventional perception. All three components help to nourish and sustain each other, but we will begin our discussion by examining the mind out of respect for its mediating role.

HEALTH
OF MIND

The great mystical traditions of the world teach that we *are* the consciousness or spirit, and that the mind is a *tool* that we use to get practical work accomplished. If we maintain a clear mind that is uncluttered by negative emotions such as fear, worry, jealousy, and anger, we are able to utilize this tool to its greatest capacity, directing it to perform positive work in all areas of our lives. However, if we allow our mind to mount a rebellion and seize the throne of higher guidance from our inner spirit, we soon run into problems.

In the next six chapters, we will examine the benefits that come from having a healthy mind and explore the best practices for keeping yours in good order.

HEALING
THROUGH JOY

chapter 1

with DR. BERNIE SIEGEL

For many, Bernie needs no introduction. He has touched many lives all over our planet. In 1978 he began talking about patient empowerment and the choice to live fully and die in peace. As a physician who has cared for and counseled innumerable people whose mortality has been threatened by an illness, Bernie embraces a philosophy of living and dying

When you are willing to reveal yourself, wounds and all, you heal yourself and everyone around you.

that stands at the forefront of the medical ethics and spiritual issues our society grapples with today. He continues to assist in breaking new ground in the field of healing. A sought-after inspirational speaker and best-selling author of _Love, Medicine & Miracles_, his new book, to be published in 2009, _Faith, Hope & Healing_, features survivor stories and his reflections on what they teach us.

T he essence of all health begins with joyful living. Joy inspires your mind, cleanses your spirit, and energizes your body. When you awaken love and laughter in your life, your mind lets go of fear and anxiety, and your happy spirit becomes the healing balm that transforms every aspect of your human experience, including your bodily health. The key is learning how to keep joy and laughter in your life, and to recognize that they are essential to your overall well-being.

For this reason, we begin our discussion of holistic wellness with Dr. Bernie Siegel, the recognized expert on maintaining your vitality and healing your body, mind, and soul through love, hope, and happiness. His insights into the role of the mind and emotions in health will change your view of the root of wellness, and his strategies for stimulating joy and laughter will give you the tools for ensuring that you keep laughter and joy in your life.

A renowned speaker and author of several best-selling books on the role of love, hope, and happiness in health and healing, Bernie has long understood the vital power of joy. He was an early pioneer in the integrative field of mind-body medicine, and he became one of the first cancer doctors to recognize that telling someone that he or she will die usually condemns the person to a self-fulfilling prophecy. Through his experiences in helping patients who face the threat of terminal illness, and through founding Exceptional Cancer Patients and its innovative mind-body counseling approach, Bernie has repeatedly witnessed how laughter and joy actually strengthen our body chemistry to heal illness and extend life. He often uses one simple phrase to sum up the power of positive emotions in health and healing: What's on your mind *matters*.

"Years ago, Norman Cousins wrote about how he overcame a significant illness by watching 'Candid Camera' and laughing," says Bernie. "He changed his body chemistry and helped himself to heal. Likewise, I know another man who was told he had a few months to live. He was a multimillionaire, and he cancelled the dress code at work and took his tie off so he could relax. He lived for another five and a half years because he began to live a more joyful life."

These anecdotes reflect the power that our thoughts and emotions wield over our physical health, as do the statistics for Monday morning death and sickness: The greatest number of heart attacks, strokes, suicides, and illnesses occur on Monday mornings when we're stressed and unhappy to be returning to our jobs. It all adds up to the same thing: When we stop feeling joy in our lives, or when we harbor long-term negative thoughts and resentments, we increase our risk of serious illness.

Can we avoid feeling negative emotions? Is it realistic to imagine that we can be happy all the time and avoid emotional pain and stress? This is not intended to be a Pollyanna-ish approach to living. We all know that life poses unavoidable challenges at times, and it isn't easy to be light and cheerful during dark moments in our lives. Even Bernie readily admits to succumbing to the pressures of work and family at different times, and having his outlook skewed by negative emotions and stress. But we can learn strategies for moving beyond pain and looking past the things we can't change.

"Most of us tend to focus on what burns us out. Years ago I kept a journal as a physician, and what I noticed was that

I focused on what troubled me all day. I remember my wife finding it and telling me that there was nothing funny in it. And I said, 'My life isn't funny.' And then she reminded me of the jokes that I used to tell her and the kids at the dinner table that had them laughing."

Just like many of his cancer patients, Bernie has also had to rediscover the simple joys of living from time to time. His experience reflects how all of us are capable of losing ourselves in the stress of our work and family routines. Consequently, the main theme behind all of Bernie's counsel is to practise self-awareness and play games to bring you back to living happily and joyfully right *now*.

As Bernie has seen repeatedly, his patients don't tend to recognize that they're mortal until they become sick, and then they rue the time they've lost. Like the multimillionaire businessman who took off his tie, we tend to not fully appreciate the value of each moment we are alive until we are threatened with losing it all. We can get past that trap by learning to live in the present—a theme we will see repeatedly among the speakers in this book—creating as much love and joy as possible in each passing instant.

To illustrate this attitude, Bernie likes to quote a comedy routine from Woody Allen in which two guys are talking, and one of them is deeply depressed. The depressed guy is talking nonstop about the bleak darkness of existence, and the other guy finally says, "What are you doing Saturday night?" The depressed guy says he's committing suicide. His friend responds, "Okay, how about Friday night?"

Despite our mortality, we can choose to live joyfully. Indeed, we *must* live joyfully. We know we won't be in our bodies forever, so we can use that awareness to spur us to refocus our attention on living in the present.

"Your life might end on Saturday, but what the hell are you doing on *Friday*? Bring some joy into your life, accept the fact that you're here for a limited time."

Why do we have trouble living a joyful life? As small children, we see the innate beauty of life and embrace the joy of living automatically. However, as we grow through childhood into adulthood, we frequently lose our vision, and we make a transition from loving ourselves to negating ourselves. Bernie has demonstrated this fact occasionally during his speaking engagements at high schools. He finds a baby and holds it up in front of the audience.

"You hold up an infant, and everybody goes 'Ooohh!'" says Bernie. "Then I grab a student that I can lift, pick him up, and everybody bursts into laughter. And I always say to them, 'What's happened in the few years in between your birth and your high school? Why do you go from being in awe of the child to laughing at yourself? Why do we become so critical?'"

Similarly, Bernie has posed another question to audiences that strikes at the heart of how we see ourselves. He asks them what we might hang in the lobby of our elementary schools, or in any of our major public buildings, that would communicate how beautiful and meaningful life is. Most people suggest butterflies, rainbows, flowers, or pictures of a baby.

"I've talked to professional trainers, who are among the most physically beautiful men and women that you have ever seen. When I ask them that, not one of them said what I consider the right answer: You hang a mirror up, so that everybody coming into the building can look at themselves and say: 'Ah, look at how beautiful and meaningful life is.'"

Somehow, in the process of growing up, we lose our ability to see ourselves as lovable and beautiful. We become increasingly self-critical and self-conscious. As newborns and toddlers we have no worries about how we look or if we appear vulnerable and "naked," but we lose this innocence as we age. Joy leaves us. Bernie is convinced that this process has much to do with the authority figures of our childhood and the messages we receive from them.

When we are children, authority figures such as parents and schoolteachers define much of our self-concept. We're fortunate when we have loving authority figures looking out for us and our emotional well-being, but if they are less tender or compassionate, we suffer wounds to our confidence and self-image that stay with us for a lifetime. Bernie recounts a story of the type of ideal caring and tenderness that we would all love to see in our authority figures.

"A teenager I know was staying at her grandmother's house, and she said to her, 'You don't have any mirrors I can really look at. There are just some small mirrors. How do I know how I look when I go to high school? I need to know.'

"In the absence of a suitable mirror, the grandmother replied: 'Come over here. Look in my eyes, and you'll see how beautiful you are.'"

As authority figures go, that's a *grand* mother. She recognized her granddaughter's need to be acknowledged, and she took the time to give her that acknowledgment in a loving, gentle, and even playful way. She affectionately coached her granddaughter through a moment of faltering self-esteem. But how many of us receive that kind of compassion and nurturing as children? Many of us don't.

As a result, we deal with issues of self-esteem throughout our lifetimes. Maybe we were criticized excessively by our parents, or perhaps even physically abused, but in general we were not taught to see our own innate beauty. Often we were drilled to see just the opposite, viewing ourselves only in negative, critical terms. As the years pass, we feel increasingly torn between these two contrary positions, still secretly wanting to feel validated, but fearful of having anyone truly "see" us.

Ironically, we are denied the opportunity to heal when we hide ourselves and our wounds. As we pull away and become emotionally remote, we become less authentic and revealing to those around us. Also, as we focus our energy on hiding ourselves, we become preoccupied instead with what others might think of us if we showed ourselves for who we really are.

This is not a healthy tactic. It may work as survival behavior in the short term, but it works against us in the long term. However, we can learn to recognize the problem and get past it. We can overcome self-denial and find joy again by learning to see ourselves clearly and developing the confidence to be our true selves. Bernie has a few techniques that he uses with patients to do this, and two that he especially likes: drawing and journaling.

Bernie's drawing exercise is a self-portrait. He has his patients draw themselves while looking in a mirror, and he tells them to try to see themselves as faultless, perfect, "divine" children. It's not necessary to be a trained artist—the idea is to simply get a loose concept of yourself down on paper where you can see it with fresh eyes.

"Draw a picture of that divine child. Then come back and look at the drawing later. Look at it as if you were looking at the picture that someone else had drawn, and ask yourself how that person feels about himself or herself? What's missing? What's exaggerated?"

The final drawing will often tell you much about your attitudes and beliefs about yourself, which can be a powerful experience. The self-portrait tends to reveal beliefs and attitudes that you're not conscious of, and your discoveries can point you toward the work that you need to do to heal your mind and heart.

Keeping a journal or diary will provide similar guidance. Journal writing tends to draw out what you are really feeling and thinking, allowing you to revisit and reflect on your inner life and perceptions as you see the words and ideas take shape on paper. As Bernie says, your life is stored within you. However, he also advises that you remember to write about joyful experiences as well, not just tragic ones, so you can regain clarity about what brings you happiness.

As you rediscover who you really are and what you really feel about the people and events in your life, you will grow in confidence and come to know what you really want and value. The next step is to summon the courage to follow your passions and your dreams.

"I remember getting a poem once that was entitled something like, 'When I Am Old, I Shall Wear Purple,' and it's about a woman who decides that when she gets old, she'll feel free enough to do all of these strange things. But at the end of the poem, she says maybe she should start practising now, so people won't think she's so strange when she gets old and starts wearing purple. And I say to everybody, if you want to wear purple, wear purple. Don't be afraid to become unique and authentic. Don't hide your uniqueness and beauty. That means your pain, too. When people ask how you are, you don't have to say 'fine' and smile. If you need help, it's okay to tell them."

Being authentic means getting past the fear of revealing your emotional wounds and your weaknesses. Some people may not feel confident or comfortable hearing your pain, and they may indeed walk away. But there will always be some who are prepared to hear you, and they will find equal solace and comfort in your company. You never need to feel ashamed of showing your wounds, and you have nothing to fear from the opinions of people who aren't interested in seeing you for who you really are.

Bernie has seen his patients make this type of shift in outlook. When they realize they're mortal and they're going to die, they discover that the things that used to bother them don't bother them anymore, including the opinions of others. Parents, in-laws, their boss at work—the negative experiences and attitudes quickly fade in importance or drop off the radar entirely. The reason is simple: If you know you're here for a limited time, you don't let circumstances and other people upset you. Similarly, if you are harboring anger or resentments, you don't stay angry at your parents or your ex-spouse for decades because of something they did or said. You learn to spend more time with the things and people you love, and less time with the things and people you don't love or who don't love you.

What happens next is almost magical: You start to let go of your past and really begin to *live* in the current moment. You can suddenly appreciate that the only moment you can truly affect or choose to enjoy is the present one. Your past is beyond your reach, and your future, as far as you know, is nonexistent. As a consequence, every moment that you're alive becomes meaningful and pregnant with opportunity for exploring your relationships and the world around you. This is a theme addressed again later in this book by people such as Jim MacLaren, Yossi Ghinsberg, Victor Chan, and Azim Jamal.

As you grow in this process, you can establish a new way of dealing confidently with the difficult challenges of your life. You can look at your work, your relationships, and your experiences and think about either changing them or changing your attitude toward them. Each situation is unique, so you have to practise discernment in what action is appropriate for that moment, but you always have choices. You can choose to leave a job or a marriage because it's not creating love and joy, or you can transform your relationship by bringing more love into it. There isn't necessarily one right answer—and there may be several solutions—but the best choice is the one that allows you *right now* to keep your sanity and your health.

Building on your increased self-awareness and restored confidence, Bernie likes to recommend strategies and playful attitudes for bringing even more richness and happiness into your life. These involve adjusting your general perception of life and events in small ways every day. One of Bernie's favorites is pretending that he has just arrived on planet Earth for the first time when he wakes up in the morning.

"I try to see everything as if it's the first time," says Bernie. "Every morning when I get up, I say to myself, 'This is your first day on the planet.' And *wow*, things get interesting.

"One morning I went to the bathroom window to see the weather outside, and the window was totally frosted over, so I got angry at the frost. I couldn't see out: I didn't know how cold it was or what I needed to wear. And then I thought, 'Hey, you're not paying attention to what you teach. It's your first day on the planet—*stop and look*.' And suddenly that window became a work of art because the crystal patterns looked like gorgeous ice ferns. It was amazingly beautiful."

Rediscovering these small, simple pleasures enriches our daily experience, but how many of us take the time to observe the beauty that surrounds us every day? Of course, you can go beyond studying ice crystals. If you take a few minutes to stop and look, you can find beauty and inspiration in hundreds of common things that you might typically take for granted. When you walk in the park or in your neighborhood, take a moment to literally stop and smell the flowers. Put your nose and your eyes up close, and study the petals and the tiny variations in color. When you have a chance to sit down outside, lean back and study the clouds, or watch the leaves moving in the breeze in the treetops, or study the flight of the birds you see, or listen to their songs. All of these simple things provide small meditations that bring you into the moment, dissolving the anxieties of the day and bringing joy and lightness into your life.

You can even look at other *people* this way. We believe that we see beautiful people, ugly people, kind people, mean people, but you can look at them like the fern patterns that Bernie describes. Rather than making superficial assumptions based on their appearance, their job title, or whether or not they are an obstacle in your path, take a moment to really look and *see* them, as you would wish they might see you. Part of this might involve trying to see *their* pain and *their* wounds, and giving some thought to what you might offer them in comfort. In this way, your own healing begins to provide healing to others, and *that's* magical as well.

Once you have a measure of self-healing under your belt, and you are reasonably comfortable with revealing yourself despite your wounds and pain, it becomes a natural and valuable progression to revisit your relationship with criticism. To be sure, you can actually benefit from a bit of constructive criticism. This is different from being a child and feeling negated by the authority figures in your life: You are now an adult who accepts that you have strengths and weaknesses in your behavior, and you are on a journey toward becoming *better*. Unconditional love notwithstanding, constructive criticism can teach you valid things about less useful aspects of your behavior, so you can improve yourself by learning to listen.

Often what we perceive to be our most difficult relationships play a vital role in that process. It could be a relationship with a family member, with a friend, with a coworker, or with a romantic partner. As we spend time together, people start to see our warts. Most of us don't like that, especially when others start to comment on their size and color, but this is an essential part of living and growing as a person. It's important that we become comfortable in recognizing our less productive behaviors, while realizing that these faults do not make us any less worthy of being on this planet. Part of the purpose of our journey is to confront them with a loving and accepting heart, and then work on improving them.

Marital partners can be an especially good source of constructive, loving criticism. No one knows this better than Bernie, who has benefited from the constructive feedback of his wife for decades. People who watch Bernie on stage and marvel at his wisdom and speaking prowess don't necessarily realize this fact. They might not appreciate that he has not always been an easy person to live with, and that he has had to do a lot of growing himself.

"One day, someone walked up to my wife after I had given a lecture and asked her what it was like to be married to me," chuckles Bernie. "And she said, 'It's a long, hard struggle.' I nodded my head in agreement."

We learn to be better people when we're strong enough to consider constructive, compassionate criticism, so it benefits us to become comfortable with it. We become better people in mind and spirit. Centuries ago, when mirrors were made of polished metal, the Sufi poet Rumi wrote that "Criticism polishes my mirror." It's a beautiful metaphor. He was saying that if you're willing to listen to criticism, you have the chance to see yourself with greater clarity and become a better human being. If we are willing to hear honest, constructive criticism from those who love us, we'll find that we've been given a tremendous opportunity to grow in wisdom and character.

"If I listen to my wife, our children, my patients, nurses, who tell me what I'm doing wrong, I don't go home saying, 'Oh, I must be the worst doctor, worst husband, worst father,'" says Bernie. "No. I know that they're telling me this because they know I care, and therefore I will change. They become my coaches."

Accepting honest criticism is also an important part of how we develop professionally in our workplace. If we aren't able to take real criticism in our work, we might seriously stunt our career growth and our financial well-being. Bernie illustrates this idea with a story about a roofing contractor who did some work on his house.

"After he was done, it rained and water came pouring in the new roof. Of course, I called him. I said, 'You know, your work, it's made it worse—I mean, water's pouring in!' He said, 'Well, your house is a problem.' I asked him to not come back. I said, 'My house wasn't a problem until *you* worked on it!'"

This is a humorous example of denial in action, but it reveals how avoiding all forms of criticism is maladaptive for growth. If you regress to a stage of denial—perhaps because you are hiding your wounds and sensitivities—you may miss valuable lessons. Furthermore, you'll likely be forced to confront the same criticism again and again until you choose to learn from it. Wisdom teaches us to learn the lesson early, so we can get on with living better. This includes getting better in our work and achieving more success in our careers.

Adults with reasonably intact self-esteem don't get upset by criticism. They know that constructive criticism polishes their mirror. Have you been given the chance to polish your mirror? If you have, what are you seeing? This is where your choices start to get interesting.

As you start to see your warts and beauty marks, achieve-ments and failures, what do you see that you would like to do differently? You have the capacity to change if you want to. Bernie thinks of it like New Year's Day: You can turn over a new leaf anytime you choose.

"You could start a New Year tomorrow if you wanted to," says Bernie. "You can't really have a new *year*, but you can become a new *person*. I think about it in the same sense that you can't have a new blackboard at the front of the class, but you can have a clean slate, so take an eraser and clean the slate.

"Yes, you've had wounds and troubles, but you don't have to keep them up there on the blackboard in front of you. Think about what you may have done in the past year, or the past day, and work on it. You can say sorry, and you can apologize, and you can let go of those who have wounded you."

Apologies are good, and so is forgiveness: Both allow us to let go of our pain and move forward. (You'll hear more about the transformational power of forgiveness later in this book with Victor Chan, executive director of the Dalai Lama Center for Peace and Education.) As you take into account any criticism that might come your way, practise letting go of resentments and grudges that you hold toward people who have hurt you. This will release you from negative emotions that weigh you down and prevent you from living joyfully.

In this process, you might even find it helpful to practise a little selective memory. You'd be surprised how easy it is to move forward and live happily when you simply forget things that, as painful as they may have been, simply have no direct bearing on your present life and circumstance. Bernie had such an experience thrust on him unwittingly, and it taught him a huge lesson about forgiving and forgetting.

"A few years ago I fell off the roof, hit my head on the pavement, and developed amnesia. It was wonderful because I'd get up with no memory of the past. Everything was beautiful and new. . . . My wife and I got along beautifully. I had no trouble with the kids."

Bernie quips that once his memory returned, he had to go and see a therapist! His point, expressed with typical humor, is that you can save yourself a lot of pain and suffering by cultivating an ability to move on from the things that really don't directly affect your present.

With the power of choice, you can choose to reinvent your life and pursue the attitudes, outlooks, relationships, and situations that are important to you *now*. As Bernie says, you can approach it as if it were New Year's Day with a new set of life resolutions.

"Keep seeing each day as the beginning of a new year. It's okay to make resolutions. It's restarting yourself, rebirthing yourself, re-parenting yourself. You don't have to wait for January 1 to start again. You can start today."

Bernie has seen how people are emotionally and spiritually reborn when they learn they have limited time left to live, but *you* don't have to wait until you have a terminal disease. You can think about how to "save your life" right now. You can make meaningful changes by beginning a new year and a new life. Is there something you dream of doing? What is stopping you from doing it *now*? You may have more resources at your disposal than you realize.

"Where do you want to live? What job do you want? All of these things are significant. Don't wait until somebody gives you a limited time to move to Colorado or Florida or wherever you want, or to take a different job, pick up your violin, and leave your law office. It can be really fun. On New Year's Eve when you know you're going to wake up tomorrow and start a new life, you're going to go to bed and have a good night's sleep."

Shrug off the weight of your old habits, release yourself from fears of being "seen," and enter a new world of wakefulness, where you feel gratitude for every opportunity you have to meet life in the present moment, for better or for worse. Like the patterns in the ice crystals, you can make your life an experience of richness and vitality.

Your own New Year's Day is the beginning of adopting a new attitude and behavior for living with laughter, love, and vitality. From your new childlike orientation toward life, you can adopt a playful spirit for every moment of your life and begin creating joy in every situation. To understand how this works, consider some of the things that Bernie has done in the most mundane circumstances: For starters, imagine making your *own* holiday for yourself and your kids.

"Make your own holidays. What would be so terrible if you said to the kids, 'Hey, this Monday, you don't have to go to school. We're taking a holiday for the family.' I'll bet you get a big grin out of them. Do something that's just fun. They'll never forget it.

"If you run a business, what if you said to everybody, 'Hey folks, no work today. We're all just going to enjoy each other.' They're going to work harder for you than if you made them work every day and never gave them a holiday."

Inventing holidays is a tool for creating more joy on even the most ordinary day. It's all part of Bernie's general approach that he calls "waking up the child" in you.

"Life is difficult, but how about waking up the child in you and finding a little humor? I drove some teachers crazy during a school visit because I said to the kids, 'Hey, do you ever see a sign, "Wet Floor" in the hallway?' And they all replied, 'YES!' So I said, 'Do you ever do it?'"

It's life-affirming fun: Take life literally, and have a chuckle with it.

"If you see a sign 'Wet Floor,' go ahead and do it. I walk into places where it says nobody's allowed, and I just say to the guards, 'I'm a nobody.'"

Becoming childlike is intrinsic to becoming more joyful. You might not be understood by the people around you, but what's the alternative? Trudge around with a grim expression just so others will take you seriously? If that's what it takes to gain respect, then reconsider whether or not you want to be "respectable." Joy and laughter are more fun and healthier. As Bernie shows, the world becomes a different place when you approach it like a child.

"I was in a lineup once, with about six or eight people in front of me. The woman helping everybody said, 'All right, dear, what is it?' So I walked right up to the front of the line and started telling her what I needed. Of course, everyone's wondering, what the hell is he doing? But they're afraid to speak up and interrupt me, so I turn to them and I say, 'Oh, you know I'm her boyfriend, so when she said "dear," I thought she was talking to me.' They all smiled and let me go. The woman knew I was being a nut, so she didn't say a word until the next day. She told me they were all asking, was I her husband or her boyfriend?"

Can you see yourself doing this in public? It's a great way to exorcise your self-conscious respectable ego while bringing healing laughter into your life. People could be laughing with you or *at* you. Is that a terrible thought to face? People laughing at you? Give that one some thought. If you discover that this idea frightens you, spend some time looking in the mirror again so you can remember who you are. If you know who you truly are, then no amount of laughter at your expense could ever hurt you, yet that same laughter could be a teaching device and healing balm for everyone around you, including your children.

"Let the healthy, fun-loving personality out," says Bernie. "And if you teach it to your kids and embarrass them regularly, they'll lighten up and live a different life also."

Being childlike brings you fully into the moment, and when you're in the moment, the fears and worries of the past and future automatically drop out of your consciousness. The joyful energy and lightness that follow provide a healing balm not only for you, but for all those around you.

Are you ready to bring new joy and love into your life? Pick the day and start a new year and a new way of being. Regardless of whether or not we are the picture of health, all of our days are numbered: We never know when we'll draw our final breath. As one man with cancer told Bernie, "Time isn't money—it's *everything*." Or as Dean Martin cheerfully remarked to Frank Sinatra (or was it the other way around?), "Always live each day as if it were your last—and one day you'll be right!"

So take a walk today. And as Bernie says, when you see a flower, reflect if that were the last flower you were ever going to see, how would it affect you? Too many people wait until they have a life-threatening illness before they wake up and start seizing the precious moments that life gives them. You don't have to. You can consciously choose to invigorate your life by addressing your fears, healing your wounds, and reconnecting with your playful child self. We are *all* dying people, so take time and indulge yourself with some of the games and techniques that Bernie offers. Get into the practice of knowing yourself, learning to love the child that you are, and not being afraid of showing yourself to the world. When you are willing to reveal yourself, wounds and all, you heal yourself and everyone around you.

It could save your life because as Bernie says, what's on your mind *matters*.

FINDING TRUE HAPPINESS

chapter 2

with DR. STEPHEN POST

Dr. Stephen Post is director of the Center for Medical Humanities, Compassionate Care, and Bioethics in the School of Medicine at Stony Brook University. He has spent years studying what makes us truly happy, and is the coauthor of one of the definitive books on the subject, *Why Good Things Happen to Good People*. Outside the classroom, he is also

In times of darkness, somehow we find the seeds for greater victory.

president of the Institute for Research on Unlimited Love (IRUL), a nonprofit organization founded in 2001 through the philanthropy of the John Templeton Foundation and dedicated to the funding of research into the roots of altruism and compassion.

If you are finding fresh laughter every day, you are well on your way to being as happy as any of us could ever hope to be in this often troubled world. Happiness is the magical elixir we all seek at the heart of living and, as Bernie Siegel points out, being happy and joyful is powerful medicine. Research has shown that laughter decreases stress hormones and improves our immune system, and that happy emotions may be the most reliable form of cold and flu prevention. The lesson: If you want to improve your health in body and mind, learn how to practise the true pursuit of happiness.

But what makes us really happy? There's no simple checklist for "acquiring" happiness, but we can start by eliminating what does *not*. A couple of years ago, I was asked to moderate an expert panel of leading social thinkers and researchers on the nature of true happiness, sponsored by the Dalai Lama Center for Peace and Education. They presented an idea that I found deeply reassuring. Beyond the basic essentials of food, water, clothing, a secure night's sleep, and a safe place to live—and they had research to back this up—no amount of money can make you exponentially happier.

If you also find that idea reassuring, or if you have ever wondered about how to create lasting happiness in your life, you might enjoy what Dr. Stephen Post has to say on the subject.

I had Stephen on *The Good Life* show twice in 2008, before and after he made his way to Sydney, Australia, to participate in the third annual "Happiness and Its Causes" international conference. This enormous event drew over 4,000 participants and included dozens of speakers ranging from the Dalai Lama to happiness researchers, professors, writers, and thinkers such as Stephen. In the course of our interviews, he shared some of the insights from that conference, as well as the research into what truly makes us happy.

I'm going to save you some time right now, in case you're in a rush, and I'll give you the answer straight up. Are you ready? Brace yourself. The big secret: We find happiness by helping others.

Are you kidding? What about the new car? What about vacations in the French Riviera? What about a full bank account? Hair like Brad Pitt or Angelina Jolie?

Sorry, but the research shows that none of that stuff really strikes at the nub of true happiness. The fact is that beyond the basics of food, shelter, physical safety, and companionship, we actually get the greatest and most lasting satisfaction when we help other human beings. This idea continues to show up in scientific studies, with researchers recording it with psychological testing, questionnaires, and even EEGs and MRIs. Basic happiness is fulfilled when we satisfy our elemental needs, but beyond those essentials, the things we tend to pursue in an effort to become happier are proven *not* to increase joy.

"There's a set point for happiness that is reached when people climb out of frustration and anxiety and stress due to concerns about where that next meal is coming from—they *are* happier," says Stephen. "But beyond that—the $200 pair of designer jeans, the extra cars, the new video games for the X-Box—they do not make people happier."

Stephen likes to point to graphic examples in which money and wealth are not the final word on happiness. For example, Americans reported greater levels of happiness in 1936 than today. Consider that for a second. Our average level of material wealth, with stereos and cars and all the rest, is vastly greater today than it was in 1936, yet we are *less* happy as a society.

"That was the tail end of the Depression. Jimmy Braddock was the heavyweight champion of the world and a third of Americans were using outhouses. I'm not suggesting that if we all get rid of our plumbing and buy outhouses, that will make us happy, but I will suggest that when we had less, life was a little simpler, and yet we were happier."

You can probably relate personally to this idea. Early in life, most of us experience the struggle of earning starting wages and trying to make ends meet, yet this is also a time of incredible growth and awakening. Life is rich with prospects and possibilities, and your ability to survive independently is its own profound reward. Surprisingly, you are "happy" despite living with relatively low income. Where do we look then to increase our happiness, if not along the traditional lines of financial wealth, luxury, and rewards? If we accept the basic tenet that happiness is generated by experiences beyond monetary gain, the next obvious question is: What are those outside experiences, and how do we create more of them?

Our mental state regarding money and happiness is well documented, particularly regarding the effects of charitable giving. Stephen points to a large study that was done between the University of British Columbia and Harvard Business School and reported in *Science*. They discovered that in fact money *can* buy you happiness—if you *give* it to someone else.

"When people contribute philanthropically and charitably to others, their self-reported happiness is much higher compared to those who don't. The research also looks at businesspeople who receive bonuses: Again, those who receive bonuses and give significantly to others report far more happiness."

If there is still a part of you that wants to believe that "Those who say money can't buy you happiness don't know where to shop," consider some more research that proves the opposite. The National Institutes of Health in 2006 took 19 subjects into a laboratory and gave them a checklist of charities. They asked the subjects to think about either donating a sum of money to charity or keeping it for themselves. Using magnetic resonance imaging to monitor their brain activity, they then asked the subjects to place a checkmark next to the box of the charity they would like to donate to.

"When they check the box, a part of their brain lights up," says Stephen. "Technically, it's called a mesolimbic pathway, but forget that. It's the deep emotional part of the brain that is associated with joy and happiness, and it even doles out feel-good chemicals like dopamine and serotonin, the very things that we're using to treat depression.

"Here we have a brain picture of what's always been called the 'helper's high'—the sense of buoyancy, of warmth, of well-being, of physical health—that is associated with even low thresholds of volunteering. There is something about connecting with this part of the human essence that actually is good for us in terms of the health, the happiness, even the longevity of our lives."

Clearly, we are hardwired to be happy when we give. This idea won the day and actually made it into the major media outlets at the 2008 Sydney conference. The *Sydney Morning Herald* published a wrap-up front-page newspaper article, which essentially said that the key to happiness is doing unto others. Now that's a message that people from every tradition on the globe recognize.

One of the best debates at the Sydney happiness conference pitted Marty Seligman from the University of Pennsylvania against Dan Gilbert of Harvard. These two well-known happiness professors have essentially opposite views on the nature of what makes us happy. Looking at their discussion, you catch a glimpse of the spectrum of current intellectual thought on what comprises happiness.

"Gilbert is famous for saying that having kids doesn't make us happier," says Stephen. "I disagree with that. Gilbert's definition of happiness is basically hedonic: It is about pleasure in the moment. And, of course, if that's your full definition of happiness, then all you're experiencing in parenthood are diapers, 36-hour days, and making formula all night while your own needs and gratification sit on the back burner.

"On the other hand, Seligman sees happiness as having three major elements. First—and this is not the most important; in fact, it's the *least* important—is hedonic pleasure. Second is immersion, or full engagement. Seligman and Csikszentmihalyi, the famous psychologist who wrote the book *Flow*, talk about this. Total immersion in what you're doing is a kind of happiness. Finally and most importantly is meaning or nobility of purpose—having some kind of pursuit in life that really is contributing to the world around you.

"It turns out that people who have that higher form of happiness—that deeper sense of flourishing—actually get more joy hedonically. They take more pleasure out of the simple gifts of life; they get more delight out of a burning log or colors in the leaves. And, in my view, this ties together to make one important message about happiness: *It's simple to be happy; it's difficult to be simple.*"

That little couplet was the theme of Stephen's presentation in Sydney. To illustrate the joy of simplicity, he points to the qualities and characteristics of his favorite historical "happy" people who found lasting contentment in their lives: the Buddha, Walt Whitman, Baruch Spinoza, and others.

"There is really a lot to be said for simplicity," says Stephen. "I don't mean that we need to go without and suffer the challenges of life when our basic needs are unmet, but fundamentally there is beauty in simplicity, and it is related to happiness. To be uncluttered, to be open to the novelty of the moment, is a beautiful thing."

Practising simplicity and generosity are wonderful ways to promote a happier life, but lasting joy is also tied to the concept of resilience. Stephen's organization, the Institute for Research on Unlimited Love, funded a study in California on resilience and stress through the Department of Veterans Affairs medical system for soldiers returning from Iraq. Through their research they've shown that some people respond to catastrophic and traumatic events by going into post-traumatic stress syndrome, while others are able to work through their hardship and pain to emerge with a greater sense of meaning, humanity, and com-passion. So the question is: Why do some people navigate these kinds of experiences with resilience while others don't?

"One of the most significant factors is the extent to which an individual has experienced tender, loving care in family life. The amount of empathy in their family history matters, as well as whether or not they have had non-parent mentors. Mentors can teach us how to stumble upon the joy of happiness through giving, so there is a relationship between giving, happiness, and getting through the deserts of life."

Another aspect of trauma recovery comes down to the simple choice of the individual. For example, during grief counseling, there comes a moment when no matter what's happened, you have a choice to make: Either get more bitter, or get better. Many people will experience low points in life—disappointments, catastrophes, terrible medical diagnoses—bad things happen to us all. But the question is: Can we rise above it? And can we even go so far as to create beauty and love in the wake of disaster and defeat?

"Take, for example, Dan Gottlieb, a psychologist from Philadelphia. He was in a traffic accident, and wound up quadriplegic, paralyzed for life. While he was in the rehab hospital, the question on his mind was: How can I kill myself?

"Then, one evening, a night nurse came along. She said, 'Dr. Gottlieb, I have a question. I've been thinking about taking my own life. Does everybody get to that point at some stage?' Gottlieb said, 'Sit down and talk about it.' He listened to her attentively with love and respect, really hearing her for about an hour. She walked away feeling greatly relieved, but he also had a realization. He discovered that he could live life as a quadriplegic because he could help other people—he could be a listener.

"He now has an NPR show called 'Voices in the Family.' People call from every nook and cranny of North America to talk to Dan Gottlieb because he makes them feel that whatever their concerns are, they are significant, their lives are special, and they are worth hearing."

Another stirring example of resilience is the story of Howard Lutnick, the CEO of the New York trading firm Cantor Fitzgerald, which lost almost 700 people at the World Trade Center attack. While watching him interviewed in 2007, I was deeply moved by his personal story of recovery after the loss of about two-thirds of his employees, including his own brother. First of all, he chose to build back the company. Secondly, he focused much of the renewed enterprise on *giving* back by providing for the families of Cantor Fitzgerald employees killed in the 9/11 attack. How many of us can imagine recovering from the grief and trauma of such an event and managing to stay focused on philanthropy? It's another of those stories that amazes and inspires me—how in times of darkness, somehow we find the seeds for greater victory. Stephen has also looked into recovery and resilience around 9/11.

"We funded the big study that looked at the extent to which a catastrophic situation like 9/11 brings out our capacities for compassion and love. We all saw that people had turned to each other as neighbors and held out their hands. They were consoling one another, expressing kindness and generosity in ways that otherwise they'd been too busy or too caught up to do, but does that change stick with them?

"It turns out that about a third of those individuals who felt a kind of transformation around 9/11 really did change their lives, and they are now pursuing different kinds of vocations and activities in life. So for about a third of people, catastrophic events shake them out of the routines of their lives, the routines that otherwise keep them focused on self-centered goals."

This leads us to the heart of the matter: What might it take for each of us to have that kind of a shift in perspective? We are capable of learning to act compassionately and appreciating the richness of our lives without traveling to hell and back. However, we have difficulty maintaining a compassionate perspective. We live in a society that for the last half century has been based on principles that do not promote peace and simple contentment, individual or cultural. Through a regular bombardment by television and other media, we have been taught (and we teach our children) that bigger is better, and that life has winners and losers. We see it in our consumer culture and business enterprise with the struggle to be number one: McDonald's has to beat Burger King; Coke has to triumph over Pepsi. This attitude has translated itself into our community and personal relationships, where competitive thinking fuels antagonism between individuals. We live in a turbo-charged capitalist culture where we even drive around with bumper stickers: "He who dies with the most toys is the winner." Quite simply, this kind of thinking doesn't promote social harmony, generosity, or happiness, especially for our kids.

"One of the worst things we can do is to overindulge our children. We love them wrongly if we create complacency and irresponsibility, and also create a sense of self-worth in our kids that is founded on material possessions and not on qualities of character and goodness. And that is happening, it is being studied, and it is a fact.

"It doesn't mean that there aren't wonderful kids growing up in our society today—there are. But there's a whole other group that is more materialistic than we've ever seen in the past, and that is *not* enhancing happiness for our kids. In fact, depression rates and anxiety are sky-high among youth."

The challenge today, more than at any other time in history, is for our kids to learn the joy of living simply. This is a hurdle, given the age in which they live, and we don't often make it easier for them.

"It's the extra pair of designer jeans. It's the $25 skateboard hat that you pick up online. The kids collect 15 or 20 of them, parents permitting, and they just fill a shelf in the hallway. Where does it end? You go from one iPod to another. It gets a little fancier and a little fancier, and every time the improvements come along, everybody wants to get whatever it is. Meanwhile we're not learning how to love one another—how to be generous, how to be creative, how to be compassionate. We're not learning the kind of joy that comes from the simple, good life."

How can we encourage that kind of happy simplicity? All we have to do is get out of the way of it! Yale University conducted a study that was published in 2007 in the journal *Nature*. Researchers took over 200 10-month-old toddlers who could not yet speak, and showed each of them a simple puppet show that featured three characters. In it, puppet number one attempts to climb up an incline, but can't get to the top and falls down. Puppet number two, the "Good Samaritan," comes along and helps puppet number one up the incline. Then the third puppet, Mean Jack, appears and pushes puppet number one back down.

Here's the punch line: The researchers then take the three puppets, which are all the same color, just slightly different in shape, and present them to each toddler in turn. Eighty-five percent of the toddlers reach out and grab a puppet. *Ninety* percent of those who grab a puppet pick the Good Samaritan.

"That tells you something about human nature. There is an innate delight that comes from acts of kindness and goodness, even from just observing kind and good acts. And it turns out that even infants as young as a year and a half— and this is *well* established—can actually engage in active compassionate activity. For example, they will intervene and call an adult in when one of their little peer toddlers is hurt, so there's a lot of compassion, a lot of goodness in human nature, but the question is: What buttons do we push to encourage and preserve these qualities?"

Schools may provide a special opportunity. If we want to push the right buttons, we might look at doing it in our education system where positive values can be taught and demonstrated with our children while they are still impressionable. Stephen visited one school in Australia that is following such a curriculum, the Geelong Grammar School.

"They have a wonderful new project on Positive Psychology and it looks like it's going to be generalized across all of Australia in a really creative way. The focus is on gratitude, forgiveness, compassion, respect, awe, optimism, and so forth—positive emotional states. Students learn about practising these attitudes. They write about their experiences, journal, and reflect on great philosophers and thinkers who have had something to say about these kinds of human assets. The curriculum is a kind of education of the heart, and it's something very similar to what the Dalai Lama Center wants to do in the Vancouver area."

Educating the heart—it strikes me as a beautiful idea that we could do this in a systematic way through our schools. You can also start this process in your own home with your family. You might start with simple family discussions about values, or you might decide that you want to look for further guidance in religious teaching. The goal is the same. If we can learn how to express positive emotions and attitudes in our daily living, starting even in small ways, we can garnish more of the fundamental happiness in our lives that researchers like those at the U.S. National Institutes of Health have seen in their study on charitable giving.

It's never too late to get engaged in thinking and talking about positive values and what you can do to encourage happiness and generosity in your life. You can get started now. You can begin by practising compassion and charity in your own household with those closest to you, and watch the transformation that happens when you treat your children, your spouse, your partner, your siblings, your parents with simple, consistent kindness and service. Then take this same practice of compassion and service into your community around you. Look at giving something of yourself where help is needed, whether it's through volunteering with an organization or making a financial donation to a worthy cause. And as you do this, you may be amazed at how your own feelings of happiness and contentment change.

"The best of us emerges when we have the kind of purpose, the kind of intentionality that Aristotle talked about. We never really know if we're happy in life until our last breath, until that moment when we are able to look back and see that we lived meaningfully."

CHOOSING TO LIVE

chapter 3

with JIM MacLAREN

Jim MacLaren is a motivational speaker, author, and founder of the philanthropic Choose Living Foundation. His personal struggle to overcome crippling injuries has shaped his inspirational outlook on

The world is starving for spirit; we need to be reminded that life is an amazing opportunity, regardless of our circumstances.

what it means to enjoy the gift of life. He is a graduate of Yale University and a recipient of the Arthur Ashe Courage Award in 2005.

Living with joy and finding the simple peace and happiness that Dr. Bernie Siegel and Dr. Stephen Post describe is tough for many of us. Sometimes our optimism and positive attitudes take a beating even before we get out of bed in the morning. How many of us find ourselves dreading the day and wishing we could just go on sleeping? Not so much tired in body, but tired in spirit? Maybe our lives feel humdrum and routine. Work can feel unrewarding, marriages worn out, and our children a constant challenge. Some part of our brain wonders how we got here.

If you're like most of us at the dawn of the 21st century, you've probably been touched at one moment or another by this sense of despair. You've asked why we're here, and you've questioned the purpose of our lives. In these moments, regardless of our efforts to maintain the joy that is foundational to our mental, emotional, and spiritual health, it feels difficult to keep striving. We feel stuck.

That's why I'm thankful for the wisdom of Jim MacLaren. When I need inspiration to overcome obstacles or setbacks in my own life, I think of Jim. For me, he is the supreme example of perseverance and determination to get back up again when life knocks you down. He has faced personal challenges in his lifetime far larger than anything most of us ever will, and he has come through them with an inner strength that is truly incredible. To understand what I mean, you have to know Jim's story.

It starts promisingly enough. In the early 1980s, Jim was a 300-pound linebacker playing for the Yale University football team. After finishing his undergraduate degree, he decided to take a year to study theater in New York City. He was young, good-looking, athletic, happy, and in the prime of his life.

Then suddenly, three weeks into his program in the fall of 1985, he was felled by a violent and catastrophic accident. While riding his motorcycle home from a rehearsal one evening, he was hit by a 40,000-pound bus on Fifth Avenue and 34th Street. He was thrown 90 feet, his body left crumpled on the pavement, lungs ruptured, most of his ribs broken, and his spleen and liver damaged. The police chalked his body on the street, and the hospital declared him "dead on arrival."

I feel chills when I try to imagine the scene of the accident. All of us have probably had a close escape, narrowly avoiding a serious accident at some time in our lives, and Jim's accident is like our worst nightmare. But he was also the subject of a small miracle: Medical staff discovered Jim was still barely alive. Finding a faint pulse, they rushed him into an operating room, and after 18 hours of surgery, they were able to stabilize him in his comatose state. When he eventually awoke eight days later, he was missing his left leg below the knee. He was disoriented and had no recollection of the eight days since the accident, but he was grateful to be alive.

He now had a significant personal challenge. Apart from the fact that he would never play competitive football again, he had to deal with weeks and months of physical rehabilitation to return to some semblance of his former physical self using his new prosthetic leg. He would miss the first semester of his theater program while he was in a New Jersey physical rehabilitation center. All the while, he would have to fight through the pain on his way back to being mobile again.

"I only had the one leg, but I would get on the inclined bench every day," says Jim. "I would judge my recovery by the amount of tears that lessened each time. I did squats, worked, and sweated until the physiotherapists just couldn't believe it."

Incredibly, Jim managed to return to classes for the second semester of his theater program in early 1986, albeit with still frequent physiotherapy sessions and much pain in his body.

"Then in that spring of 1986, I auditioned again for the Yale School of Drama, and I was one of 15 who were accepted. I started the following fall of 1986, but things were very painful. I was still very heavy, an ex-football player, which made the rehabilitation incredibly tough."

The physical shock of Jim's accident was immediate, but the full extent of the emotional shock took one year to surface.

"The real depression hit me around the one-year anniversary of my accident. I lifted up the sheet, and I saw my leg. I said, 'Oh my God, this is me for the rest of my life.'

"I left school. I abandoned a work-study assignment, and I went to New York to hit the bars with my friends. When I got back to the school, I was called into the office of the dean, Earle Gister, who's a famous director and arguably ran the finest drama school in the world. He looked at me and said, 'First of all, you're on probation. Look, you've got to be a professional. You can't shirk your responsibilities.' And then like a true father figure, he took his glasses off and said, 'Now what can I do for you?'

"It was that day that I walked into the gym at Yale and got into the pool, even though it was difficult and painful to take my prosthesis off. I was a 300-pound rock with arms, but I started swimming. And as soon as I got in the water, I thought, 'My God, I'm moving. I'm back in life.'"

Jim was fortunate to have a number of good friends who gave him emotional support all this time. As he slimmed, trimmed, and gained improved mobility, they even encouraged him to consider new alternatives in sports. Triathlon and ironman competitions were growing in popularity, and new attention was being given to disabled athletes in all sorts of sports. Jim came across a book on triathlons at the library that captured his imagination, and his friends gave him magazines with stories describing marathon runners and triathletes who were competing with one leg.

He suddenly saw a new vision for himself. Here was an avenue where he might focus his physical, mental, and spiritual energies and transcend the blow he had been dealt. He began training, trimming, and toning his physique to become a competitor in events that would eventually include the New York City Marathon and the Ironman Triathlon in Hawaii. After having started swimming simply for rehabilitation, and then bicycling because it was painful to walk to class with his prosthetic, he was now en route to becoming a marathon runner and triathlete. It was Jim's first big lesson of his recovery: Engage yourself in life by choosing the path of action and hope, regardless of how enormous the obstacles might seem.

"Starting from a place where I really just wanted to see what I could do, I became the world's fastest human being on one leg," says Jim. "I was competing only against able-bodied athletes, and I guess I got noticed because I was beating 70 to 80 percent of the two-legged athletes."

He set dozens of records, and regularly finished ahead of 80 percent of his competitors. As a triathlete and marathon runner, I can tell you firsthand that is an incredible achievement. To this day, I believe Jim still holds the world record for the fastest one-legged Ironman time. He was traveling all over the world, and he added motivational speaking and mentoring to round out what was becoming a very successful career.

It's an amazing story, right? Unfortunately, I've told you only the preamble.

In 1993, Jim experienced the blow that would create the greatest challenge in his life. During a triathlon in Mission Viejo, California, a race marshal on the cycling course segment misjudged the speed of the oncoming cyclists and waved a truck into Jim's path at an intersection. Jim hit the truck at full speed, and the impact catapulted him from his bicycle into a signpost. When he awoke in hospital, the doctors told him the grim news. He had broken his neck, and would never move his limbs again. He was a quadriplegic.

I cried when Jim told me this in our first interview. What would you do at that point? As Jim says, he didn't know if he had the ability or even the desire to try to recover a second time, especially against such a profound physical handicap. He was staring at life and death, inasmuch as he had understood life to that point.

"It was a whole new plane of existence," says Jim. "When I lost my leg, I was at a rehabilitation center where all my friends were quadriplegic and paraplegic, so I had a little bit of a window into what it was like, but basically, you can't know what it's like until it happens to you."

He was lucky at that point to have a friend who became a catalyst for his most dramatic recovery.

"Even a mentor needs a mentor, and I was very fortunate at that time to have a mentor that got me to deal with this one key fact: The word 'why' does not matter. Why it had happened wasn't important because I still had to get up every day."

Jim began the long process of a second physical rehabilitation, and this time the process lasted half a decade, but he stunned everyone.

"I had the pain and the logistical aspects of four to five hours getting ready, getting between the bathroom, and getting dressed, and getting helped every day, but truly, once I made the decision to engage life, all those logistics became very peripheral."

To the astonishment of many in the medical profession, he started to regain some movement in his limbs, an incredible achievement in itself, even if it wasn't enough to walk again. All the while, he wrestled with the purpose and value of his life.

"Although I went through the ups and downs of it, the ultimate decision through all of it was what I call 'Choose Life'—engage *life* at every single moment."

By engaging life, Jim means that we need to recognize that the current moment is the only one we can act on. The past cannot be changed, and consequently the "why" of our situation is not as important as what we do to change it.

Since his realization, he has only grown in his conviction that being alive is a gift, and life is worthwhile for its own sake. Jim has taken his own experience and learning, drawn strength from the example of others who have mentored and inspired him, and continues to tour as a sought-after motivational speaker while also working as a mentor and life coach for others. He teaches people how to engage life with complete conscious awareness and decisive action in every moment, and his mentoring helps them to apply this type of awareness and courage in the face of whatever particular circumstances confront them.

One of his simple techniques for dealing with challenging circumstances involves how you wake up in the morning.

"When I speak to people about their own lives, I talk about that ethereal period when we first wake up," says Jim. "That period when we're not quite awake, and we're not quite asleep—we just *are*. We don't owe money yet, we're not fat yet, I'm not even in a wheelchair yet. Instead of hitting the snooze alarm, I try to get people to think of something that makes them feel deeply good about themselves. What you imagine in that moment becomes a tool you can use for the rest of that day. When you feel overwhelmed or afraid, you don't need to go over in the corner and meditate like a buddha. You can be in the middle of a board meeting or in the middle of a class, and recapture that moment, that five minutes in the morning when you felt good about yourself. It's a powerful tool to reconnect with your inner self, the source of real happiness."

Jim's inspirational courage, determination, and mentorship gained public recognition at the 2005 ESPY Awards. On that special night in Los Angeles, Oprah Winfrey presented him with the Arthur Ashe Courage Award, together with Emmanuel Ofosu Yeboah, the young one-legged Ghanaian man who cycled across Ghana to raise awareness for disabled people. The link between them: Emmanuel was riding a bicycle purchased with a grant from the Challenged Athletes Foundation, the organization originally founded to help Jim following his second accident.

During the presentation of the award, Oprah made a verbal reference that would provide the next catalyst in Jim's inspirational work. By pure happenstance, Oprah echoed Jim's personal motto when she introduced them.

"Oprah said 'Emmanuel and Jim chose life.' There was a 10-minute standing ovation. They were not to be quieted."

The synchronicity of her choosing that phrase, and the resonating sound of those familiar words, told Jim he had to do something. Following the ESPY Awards ceremony, he established the Choose Living Foundation, an organization dedicated to fund-raising and volunteer efforts to help children, adults, and families in adverse circumstances to overcome the obstacles that prevent them from fully participating in life.

"Choose Living came from the magic of that night. I don't know how else to describe it, except that the kernel of the foundation began that night when Hollywood forgot who they were for 10 minutes. No one was posing. They just cried, and I cried, and Oprah cried, and Emmanuel cried, and that's how Choose Living was born. There was just so much magic that I thought *I need to start a foundation.*"

And you can't imagine a more ambitious or important mission statement than the one Jim established for the Choose Living Foundation.

"The mission statement is spread love and compassion throughout the universe, whether it's through inspiration, or mentorship, or education, or at times financial help. We help everyone from CEOs who have addictions to kindergarten students who need someone to come and speak at their school."

Since 2005, his fund-raising and speaking schedule has grown busier, his reach has extended further, and throughout all of it he has stuck to his commitment to serve others before himself. When the producers of the "Larry King Live" show invited him to appear on the program in July 2007, the invitation put him in a bind with a prior commitment for a fund-raising dinner where he would be speaking for free. He was determined to stick to his commitment to appear at the fundraiser, so he asked Larry King's producers if they could make the timing of the interview work for his scheduled speech and get him back to the fund-raising dinner in time.

"And sure enough, they did it. They limoed me up there with my assistant Scott, and I did the show with Larry."

And when Jim arrived back at the fund-raiser, he made a happy discovery.

"All they did was extend the cocktail hour by an extra half hour," laughs Jim. "So I got there 30 minutes late, but in my opinion, the best way to get people to open up the checkbooks is to extend the cocktail hour an extra half hour. We raised a lot of money that night for the foundation."

At the same dinner, two of the friends of the man who had created the foundation spoke to Jim. Their friend, the founder, had been paralyzed from the chest down since suffering a spinal cord injury. They were unsure how to relate to him in his new condition, and they were looking for Jim's advice.

"They said, 'How do we treat him?'" recounts Jim. "And I said just love him. You know, he's the same guy. He's sitting down now, but he's still Eric, just like I'm still Jim."

Jim's wisdom and insight in seeing the true essence of people are part of what continue to inspire me about his work.

His generosity of spirit and his optimism in the face of his own struggles complete the picture. He has taken two apparently unfortunate events and used them for transformation—his own and others'. He has rubbed shoulders with celebrities such as Oprah Winfrey and Larry King, and in the process he has reached more of the world in his speaking and fund-raising. As Jim says, the world is starving for spirit, and people need to be reminded that life is an *amazing* opportunity, regardless of our physical circumstances. He has fought back from seemingly insurmountable odds to give us all a lesson in remembering the intrinsic beauty of being alive, regardless of what trials life hands us, and he has inspired and comforted thousands of people through his speaking, mentoring, and Choose Living.

Consider the lesson of Jim MacLaren's life, and make an affirmative decision to choose life every day when you awaken. Awaken your senses and your vision to see the humanity in everyone, and treat them with the compassion and kindness you would like to be shown. When you feel especially burdened in life, remember to take quiet moments to rekindle the deep peace and joy that you fostered in the early hours of the morning. If you can do that, you will be on your way to creating meaningful happiness for yourself and those you care about.

> *Our problems and our pain don't necessarily go away, but we can take the focus off of them by engaging life and appreciating the moment that life brings us with every single breath that we take.*

Wise words from my personal hero, Jim MacLaren.

SURVIVING
LIFE'S JUNGLE

chapter 4

with **YOSSI GHINSBERG**

Yossi Ghinsberg is an author and motivational speaker who was born and raised in Israel. While exploring the Bolivian Amazon during a trip to South America in 1981, he became lost in the jungle and had to survive alone for three weeks. Following his rescue,

"I discovered that there is a knowledge and a force throbbing inside me, and I realized that I knew what to do: I realized what true living is."

his experience of fighting for survival inspired him to study serious questions of existence through a variety of cultures, philosophies, and mystical practices. He is the author of *Jungle* and *Laws of the Jungle*.

J im MacLaren's incredible personal story is a triumph of mind over matter. Using pure mental determination, he has risen above the limitations of his physical body to reach great heights of personal growth and achievement in a way that we recognize as clearly heroic. But what happens when the greatest obstacle to living is our mind itself? As products of a culture that teaches us to rely on our mental impressions and calculated assessments of daily life, we often stifle our ability to experience and enjoy life as it simply appears to us each day. Rather than live in a state of alert awareness of the richness that surrounds us, we occupy our waking consciousness with incessant and burdensome thinking. In the process, we lose our connection with something even more central to living: *Being*. We become trapped in a labyrinth of mind—a jungle of thought, if you will—and we lose contact with the essence of life itself.

Yossi Ghinsberg is a teacher who has mastered life's mental "jungle" and charted the path for escaping it. Starting with a profound personal confrontation with death, followed by years of philosophical study and contemplation, he has examined the essential questions of how to cultivate a clear, peaceful mind for living in greater harmony with nature and our community around us. Similar to Jim MacLaren's transformation during his physical recovery, or the experiences of Dr. Bernie Siegel's cancer patients in facing their own mortality, Yossi's life outlook was forever changed by a dramatic experience that left him searching for meaningful answers to essential questions of being. In Yossi's case, he shows us that the primordial essence of who we truly are as human beings lies in nature, and that it is possible to reframe your mental outlook through an understanding of the natural world.

Yossi was born in Tel Aviv, and he admits he was a simple product of his culture until that day in 1981 when his life was transformed through a traumatic experience in South America. He was a young man who had grown up in a developed country, he had completed a stint of compulsory military service in the Israeli navy, and he was on an otherwise predictable path that would see him join his society in the way any of us might imagine—owning a house, a car, and working the standard "nine to five." Then he made a fateful decision when he was 22 years old to travel to South America, where he set off into the Amazon region of Bolivia, seeking adventure.

Yossi was part of a group of four travelers who decided to create their own unique trek into the Amazon. They were looking for golden riches, hidden indigenous tribes, and all the other romanticized images of jungle adventure. They never found that experience: After one month of rigorous hiking into the unknown, they began fighting among themselves over direction and leadership.

The four adventurers separated into two groups. One pair of men chose to travel up a tributary, while Yossi and another man decided to travel downriver on a raft. The two men who went up the tributary have never been seen again.

Meanwhile, the route chosen by Yossi and his partner was leading everywhere and nowhere. The river meandered for countless miles, and they had no idea where they were. Their only hope was to find human settlement and a way out of the jungle. And then their situation worsened: They suddenly found a waterfall directly in front of them. Frantically, they tried to reach the riverbank to avoid being swept over. Yossi's friend made it to the bank, but Yossi fell into the torrent of the river. Gripped by the raging current, he was swept downstream and out of sight of his desperately shouting companion.

What transpired next was as unthinkable as it was sudden. Separated from his travel mate, Yossi found himself completely alone in the jungle without a gun, knife, or any food.

"I was lost for three weeks, in the middle of the rainy season, in an environment that I did not know at all," remembers Yossi. "Israel is mainly desert, and there's no rain forest—definitely not Amazonian jungle. And my three years in the navy weren't a good preparation for survival in the forest."

Imagine being lost in the jungle, a middle-class citizen coming from the world of television, take-out pizza, and all the conveniences of modern culture. How would you face up to such a challenge? The situation drew from Yossi something of which he had no previous awareness. Facing the prospect of imminent death from starvation, disease, or being eaten by a wild animal, an inner strength he had never known before emerged.

"I had to learn to lean not on something that I'd learned, but on something that was already inside of me. This was a very, very strong awakening call for me because I realized that there is a vast pool of knowledge that goes with simply being human. I had inherited a million years of evolution. It was embedded in me, and I managed to tap into it because I didn't have a choice."

Yossi's circumstances were extreme and desperate. He was alone and isolated, without even fire for warmth. There was danger by day and night, and there was nothing else for him to do but fight for survival.

"I ate eggs that I robbed from birds' nests, I was bitten by many bugs, and once I came so close to a jaguar, I could feel its breath on my face."

Yossi was not surviving through the power of understanding or reasoning, but purely through a fundamental, existential will to live. The duress of his situation stripped him of his cultured sense of security and the self-concept that went with it. He was left with only the bare elements of what it means to be a sentient creature living moment to moment, putting him more in league with the animals of the jungle than a hotel clerk or a public accountant back in Israel.

"I survived, but not only did I survive, I even managed to thrive. I discovered that there was a knowledge and a force throbbing inside me, and I realized that when it came to it, I knew what to do. I wasn't a victim of circumstance. I found my way through action. I realized what true living is. In those moments of great danger, life was so amazing. Every minute, every day, I never had any doubts about life and my purpose because my purpose became very simple: It was to live, which is the most sacred purpose."

Yossi was found and rescued by his partner on the raft, the only other survivor from the group, who had managed to escape the jungle with the assistance of members from an indigenous tribe. Saved from the depths of the jungle, Yossi made his way back to Israel, and began to realize how profoundly he had been changed by his experience.

"When I came back home, I felt like a foreigner, even in my own home. I wondered how I could belong to such a small place when I'd been out in the world and in the rain forest, and discovered that these aspects of myself are much more universal."

The discrepancy between his sense of universal self and the constricting sense of his old identity became too much. He needed to know more, and he decided to go looking for answers.

"I left everything and I started traveling the world because I didn't have answers, but I had many strong questions that just didn't allow me to ignore them. I started discovering that whatever drives us to seek these answers is actually pushing us toward an inner exploration, and what we're looking for outside is, in reality, an inner search."

Yossi's inner search took him around the globe, and his explorations continue to this day. Since he was rescued, he has studied with spiritual teachers of different faiths and philosophies, attempting to penetrate the meaning of what he first glimpsed in the Amazon rain forest.

"I've been traveling in many different cultures, and I've been studying and searching and learning. Gradually I have created my own picture of the world, my own understanding of it."

His inner journey has taught him many lessons. He discusses some of them in his second book, *Laws of the Jungle*, in which he connects the fundamental experience of being lost in the jungle—his connection with the primordial will to live—with everything he has learned since, inspired by his travels and encounters with different people, philosophies, and mystical traditions. He has spent time in the desert with Bedouin, studied yoga, and even returned to the Amazon to live briefly with the indigenous people near the area where he was lost. All of this fulfilled his desire to learn and practise a simpler way of life than the one he had grown up with—a way of life less dominated by mind and more connected to *being*. For Yossi, the principal lesson of who we are and how we experience true peace revolves around observing and emulating the natural world's definition of being.

"The strongest influence is nature itself. To connect to nature's guidance, we observe and contemplate what *is*—the people we are, and the environment that we are."

His belief in the primacy of nature was reinforced in 1992 when he returned to the upper Amazon basin, where he had been rescued 10 years earlier. He stayed there for three years, learning about the indigenous people who had helped him, as well as reconnecting with the place that sparked his original transformation. Along the way, he helped the local people build a model ecotourism resort called Chalalán, which still thrives today.

He discovered that the simple jungle lifestyle shields a person from developing an overabundance of mental prejudices that mask the essence of what it means to be alive. The culture of indigenous people doesn't condition or distract them from actually seeing and understanding the elements of nature and their relationship with it.

"I'll give you a little example. If it's raining, most people in the city will say, 'Ah, what an awful day, what a miserable day.' That's how disconnected people are from nature. They look at rain and they say, 'It's a terrible day.' If you live in nature and it's raining, you say, 'What a blessed day.'"

What a blessing to see the earth and the land on which you depend nourished; to see the promise of a rich new harvest; to see your life and all life around you thriving. Without this connection to the natural world, rain becomes purely a discomfort and an inconvenience, something that wets our hair or muddies our clothing. Given that rain is one of many things that we have little control over, yet forms an intrinsic part of our experience, wouldn't it make sense to consciously embrace it as part of our lives?

According to Yossi, most of our anxiety and disconnection is the result of our minds' attempt to control everything that happens to us.

"If the jaguar goes hunting, and he fails to hunt, he doesn't crawl back to his den and say, 'I'm a very bad jaguar, I'm not a good jaguar. I think maybe it's my childhood experiences with my parents that have made me such a silly jaguar.' The jaguar just goes to sleep hungry and wakes up in the morning more determined. That's what nature is. Nature doesn't doubt itself. Nature is based on action.

"The only animals that need help are animals that are surrounded by us. Dogs have psychologists and psychiatrists. Cats go to see therapists. Our doubt is so contagious that we even gave it to animals. That's how unbelievable we are as a species!"

Humans are as much a part of the natural world as animals, but we have somehow lost our awareness of its fundamental principles of being. Nature expresses certain elements of randomness and chance, such as weather, but our human tendency is to insist on attempting to control everything that happens to us and around us, just as we do in our urban landscapes.

"We position ourselves within Creation, and we have separated ourselves so we think that we are actually in charge. We are not in charge. If we would only let go of that desire to control, of the shortsightedness that causes us to reach for immediate satisfaction, we'd actually see that we live in a perfect place. The place that we are part of is perfect because that place has created us."

The wisdom that grows out of Nature is the wisdom of the universe. We can attune ourselves to that wisdom if we practise stillness and listen. The animals and the plants do this all the time.

"Everbody has the ability to truly listen." There's a subtle vibration that goes through everything, and every plant, every animal is actually tuning in and receiving that information, and that's why the help you need will ultimately come from the source itself. We are part of it, but our mind is not tuned to that vibration anymore. We see ourselves as separate, but the separation is an illusion that we have created with our own minds.

"Of course, we are a very, very intelligent animal, but we live in a cage—the trap of the mind. The illusion is that we need outside help. The illusion is that we need enlightenment. There is no need for enlightenment because we *are* enlightened. We just need to surrender; we need to stop the search."

We can reconnect with nature and its innate wisdom, but an overemphasis on formal reasoning has caused us to ignore the intuitive receptiveness associated with hearing the voice of the natural world. If we aren't immediately able to gauge and measure an aspect of nature with a quadratic equation or an electron microscope, most often we're not interested or even aware of what it may be saying to us!

Yossi's remarks bring to mind other guests I've had on *The Good Life*. Not long before I spoke with Yossi, I interviewed Dan Millman on the program and we talked about the idea that there are no ordinary moments, a theme that looms large in his famous book, *Way of the Peaceful Warrior*. Yossi's definition of enlightenment follows a similar sentiment. In *Laws of the Jungle*, he says that if you ask nature for the time, it will tell you that the time is *now*.

"The time is always now; it's an eternal now. Try and grab a moment that is not now—it's impossible. Even that *now* is very hard to grab because we are living it as it unfolds."

Almost every modern-day mystic or healer will speak about this idea: Our lives are happening now, and we inhibit our experience and our joy by carrying our fears of the future and worries of the past. In following Yossi's advice and tuning in to the lessons of our natural world, we can begin to imagine a world without our neurotic egos, without the obstacles of the past and the future. We can start to take action in the now because we see nature doing this already. As Yossi teaches, nature has no problem being and acting in the now because "jaguars don't have baggage."

"There is no other species that has a concept of the past. They learn, and they use that learning for the present, but they don't carry the past as a way to drag them down. They don't look at the future as something that will interfere with the present moment as we do. We have the tendency to live in both illusionary times—past and future—while the only moment that is real life is that elusive moment that unfolds constantly."

Nature doesn't harbor feelings of being victimized; it just gets on with the business of getting things done. Have you ever stewed in anger or resentment or hurt, thinking about a wrong that you felt someone had done you? We waste so much time and energy indulging in this meaningless victim posture. It is wise and sane to recognize when you have been hurt as you need to identify the issue consciously in order to set about making new choices. However, dwelling on the idea of being a "victim" and indulging yourself in mental and emotional anguish does not advance you or improve your situation. You need to take action: In the words of Jim MacLaren, you need to "engage life." In this regard, Yossi says the creatures of nature are already *enlightened*.

If you can manage to live consciously in the moment that is the constantly emerging *now*, you enter a state of being that feels, ironically enough, like immortality.

"If you are present in that moment, you will have no worry because worry cannot be part of the now. The now can only be a response to circumstances and proper action.

"This is life. When we are talking about awakening, it's awakening to that. The moment is always now, and when the moment is always now, you're given the opportunity to respond to the moment—that's living. If you're not doing that, you're not really living. We condense our precious moments of living into worries about what we've done, and guilt and remorse, and pondering, and then desires for the future. All of this stops us from actually being here now and living."

Of course, we all have very busy minds, and a very busy culture that reinforces the idea that we cannot be satisfied in the present moment. Our culture tells us we need to acquire or achieve something that will, in turn, provide happiness for us: a new car, a new partner, a new job, a new vacation. As we pursue these things, we end up on a treadmill sprinting toward a point on the horizon that looks like happiness, but it continues to recede into the distance and we never arrive, like the "Freedom 55" financial retirement campaigns. What if your whole life was predicated on Freedom 55, and you reach age 56 without hitting it? Where does that leave you and your best-laid plans? Freedom 88?

To overcome our perceptual difficulty between seeing the natural essence of life and this artificial life of our cultural reasoning, we need to spend time contemplating nature, and perhaps even practising specialized techniques of meditation and reflection. To tear down his own perceptual barriers, Yossi spent years contemplating and observing nature, as well as peoples and cultures who live close to nature.

"When you look at people whose culture is more in tune with nature, you'll see that they have spaciousness of time. I lived in the desert with Bedouin, and I will never forget the nobility of sitting by the fire and seeing another person arrive. There would be 10 or 12 men sitting by the fire, drinking tea, speaking quietly, when suddenly another man would just approach. At that moment, the entire conversation around the fire would stop. Each one of the people in his turn would get up and greet the newcomer. That ritual would take about half an hour, just to greet somebody that came to join the sitting place. I was in awe at just how generous you can be with time.

"We have an illusion, and the illusion is that we don't have any time. Constantly we are under stress and pressure. The only thing that we have is time, and we have to celebrate and cherish that."

This reminds us of the cancer patient who told Bernie Siegel that *time is everything*. We have been given a lifetime of "time," but we fill it with so much activity and busy-ness that we exhaust any possibility of truly possessing and enjoying a few quiet moments in a day for contemplation and relaxation. It doesn't have to be that way. We can choose to slow time. We can remove many of the stresses in our daily routines and truly appreciate the moments that life brings us by practising techniques and habits that promote mindfulness and calmness. Some people meditate; some practise tai chi or yoga; some simply go walking, running, or hiking. Yossi has adopted yoga and chosen to live away from an urban setting.

Interestingly, when he travels to cities, Yossi observes that the urban environment and activity around him impacts his yoga practice.

"I do a yoga exercise every morning, and this yoga exercise starts with a breathing exercise," explains Yossi. "The breathing exercise is only eight breaths, so before I start my movement, I begin with eight full breaths. The moment that I arrive in a city and I do my morning practice, I notice my breath has changed, as if I don't even have time to breathe. And when I practise with friends of mine everywhere I go in the world, you notice that. Just focus on the breath, and see that we are in a hurry even when we breathe. There's this illusion that there's no time. We feel that we need to achieve many things, but there isn't enough time, and that actually *shortens* our time."

This anxiety—the feeling that we don't have enough time—is directly linked to our minds' desire to control everything. We feel the need to force everything to happen, to push it to happen, to *make* it happen. We don't need to make everything happen. We need to become comfortable with relinquishing control. We need to practise a special brand of acceptance for the things and experiences that life brings to us.

"We are driven by a certain need to control the elements, to manipulate the elements, to *get* out of the elements what we think we want or need. I just work on one thing—my ability to experience whatever comes, as opposed to attracting things that will make me satisfied and happy and give me what I want."

In line with Buddhist thought, Yossi is convinced that true happiness comes from simply being receptive to life and whatever it brings to us.

"I don't work on trying to get this or that. The only thing that I am working on is the ability to experience whatever life brings me. That's what I believe is the only thing that we can really do. No matter what life brings you, you can deal with it from a place of wisdom, of understanding, and of compassion."

Emphasis on wisdom: Yossi emphasizes that this kind of life orientation cannot be contrived through your intellect. You have to truly see the inherent wisdom in accepting what life brings you, otherwise you will continually struggle with your desire to control your environment, including expectations that there are certain achievements and material attainments that will make you complete and happy. It's a losing equation because either your happiness becomes contingent on material results that may or may not come to pass, or you are made miserable by receiving things or having experiences that you don't want.

"We're constantly on that pendulum. Even when we get what we want, we're already busy wanting something else.

"Why go on that equation when you can live another way? 'I will experience whatever life brings me with grace.' How about that for an equation? There's no need for control. There's nothing to push away, and there's no need to desperately attract the things we think we want. It's a ceaseless, Promethean journey, trying to control the elements."

We distort our experience through our drive to control nature and all life events. We do it through our families, our workplaces, our schools, our institutions. We separate ourselves from the reality of what is, and in the process we deny ourselves the joy of authentic being. We're shadowboxing with the illusions of our desires, and we never actually *live* the reality where we exist at this moment.

"The need to control is a burden of humanity. We say that the lion is the king of all the animals, but that is our invention. The last thing that the lion wants is to be the king of the forest. The lion likes to eat and relax—he is not trying to control anybody!"

So what happens if we cease our anxious pursuit of all the material goodies and trophies of life? We may find ourselves at the end of the "race" without much to show for our life accomplishment in the conventional way of measuring bank balances and personal net worth. Is that a terrifying thought? It's worth contemplating. What do we really take with us beyond our final breath? Yossi had an awakening about this idea when he saw a billboard on the side of a church with a message about our last shirt having no pockets, a reference to the shirt we wear in our coffin when dressed for burial.

"That shirt has no pockets whatsoever. When you think about that, you start being a businessman of life. That's what happened to me. I said to myself, I want to be a smart businessman, so let's see what investment I can make that doesn't perish. If the last shirt has no pockets, that means that all of my investments are short term because I cannot take my bank account, I cannot take my so to speak 'real estate.'

"What is it that doesn't need a pocket? What can you take with you? And the answer is the living being that I am—it doesn't need a pocket—so I decided to invest in that which is eternal. That's a smart business."

You can invest in your living being by spending some time asking yourself who you are in the deepest sense, and being prepared to make inner explorations. Too many people are looking for a quick answer outside of themselves: a pill, a guru, somebody to make them happy, but quick answers don't work. All of the big questions can be answered only within yourself. It requires years of reflection and meditation to reach those answers. This outlook runs contrary to contemporary lifestyles focused on quick results and instant gratification, but it is the only meaningful path to finding the way out of the jungle of our ego mind and its anxieties.

"There's really no other way, and this is in truth the most efficient way. Imagine your consciousness being like the physical manifestation of our world, a sphere. If you imagine that the answer is in the core of that sphere, at the center of the earth, you can see that the shortest way to reach that answer will be to drill straight underneath you: That's the shortest way. Drill *within* and you'll find it."

There's a haunting and mesmerizing paragraph in Yossi's book, *Laws of the Jungle*. It describes people living in a box, driving to their office in a boxy car, and working in a box. I read that paragraph early one morning over coffee, before my show, and it stunned me. I put the book down and I thought long about it. I felt alert and wakeful, and my wakefulness in turn made me realize: We all need to wake up. As Yossi points out, life is our greatest adventure, and we're going through it right *now*.

In our next chapter, Lynne McTaggart will describe how to further refine this mindfulness of the present moment, combining it with purposeful intention to transform physical reality for the benefit of yourself and others.

USING
INTENTION

chapter 5

with LYNNE
McTAGGART

Lynne McTaggart is an internationally recognized researcher and speaker on the science of spirituality. The author of five best-selling books, she has delved into the underlying physics of spirituality

"We are brought up with an old scientific story. We're brought up with a sense of our own separation, and yet the new science shows us we're actually part of a unity . . . and we can influence the world around us."

and nonlocal healing in *The Intention Experiment* and her giant best-selling book, *The Field*. She also teaches "Living the Field" master classes around the world, showing class attendees how to integrate the science of intention and the power of thought into their everyday lives.

What if you could think something, and then see it become reality? Recent films such as *What the Bleep Do We Know?* and popular books such as *The Secret* have looked at the idea that our thinking is capable of shaping our material reality, including the physical qualities of our own bodily health. Many practitioners of holistic medicine also talk about the power of our thoughts, but where's the proof in this idea? Where is the hard science that supports a concept that otherwise sounds merely like spooky magic? Many people talk about the power of intention in general terms, but less attention has been given to actually documenting the scientific evidence for the "miraculous" manifestations of the power of thought. Lynne McTaggart is part of a group of researchers who are changing that.

An experienced medical and scientific investigative journalist, Lynne McTaggart first touched on the power of intention while researching the scientific basis for spiritual healing and homeopathy in her best-selling book, *The Field*. While writing *The Field*, Lynne discovered that scientific studies into the physics of energy healing and prayer were taking place simultaneously all over the world. Their independent findings were encouraging—amazing in some instances. This naturally led her to the question: What might be accomplished if large groups could focus their thoughts *together* in a coordinated effort with common targets of intention?

Lynne started researching everything she could that was associated with the power of thought, including the placebo effect, but when she looked for evidence of the power of group intention, she couldn't find much.

"So I turned to my husband one night, and he said, 'Why don't you do these experiments yourself?' It sounded ridiculous to me because I'm not a scientist, though I'm a science writer."

After her initial skepticism, Lynne started to think seriously about the idea. She reflected on the fact that her best-selling book, *The Field*, was already published in 20 languages, so she knew there were readers around the world who were familiar with and excited by the concept of mind affecting matter. Could there be a way to harness this groundswell of understanding and support to conduct new research?

An idea occurred to her. Perhaps large groups of people could be organized internationally with the purpose of directing thought intentions at predetermined times and dates to targets in laboratories around the world, where scientists could then measure the effects using reliable equipment in a controlled environment. She certainly knew a lot of scientists by this point from her previous writing and research, and the Internet provided the avenue for coordinating large numbers of people in different countries and cities. If she invited readers and supporters to visit a website dedicated to the experiment, perhaps she could direct them to perform large-scale thought experiments as an online community of intention senders. It was an idea that could work, and she seized on it.

Lynne began organizing with her contacts in the scientific community, and very soon she had the beginnings of what would famously become known as The Intention Experiment. Since March 2006, she and a group of laboratory scientists have conducted regular trials in which they ask participants, via a dedicated website, to direct their mental intentions to targets around the world. The project has involved physicists and psychologists from the International Institute of Biophysics in Germany, Cambridge University in England, Princeton University, the University of Arizona, Pennsylvania State University, and the Institute of Noetic Sciences in the United States. Their first experiment was modest in that it involved a mere 16 people in London sending identical, scripted healing thoughts to four simple targets at a laboratory at the International Institute of Biophysics in Germany: two types of algae, a jade plant, and a human subject. Since then, the experiments have grown vast in scope, involving thousands of people around the world, who access the website at predetermined dates and times to view targets and read instructions for their latest mental intention experiment.

So what have they found? At first glance, the results might not look earth-shattering, but the implications are enormous.

In the first experiment using 16 experienced meditators in London, Lynne showed them images of the target subjects in Germany on a computer screen. Then she showed them a sentence to describe their healing intention in words, which she also read aloud to them, so that all 16 intention senders would be sending exactly the same thought. Meanwhile, in Germany, the laboratory researchers used extremely sensitive equipment to take measurements around the actual intention targets for biophoton emissions, the tiny amounts of low-intensity light that are emitted by all living things. An increase in biophoton emissions is generally measured when an organism is stressed, so the research group created a situation where each target organism would be biologically stressed, and the intention-sending subjects would then attempt to lower their biophoton counts. To create the stress conditions, the researchers put a pin through a leaf of the jade plant, added vinegar to one of the algae varieties, and gave the human target three cups of coffee.

"We were simply trying to show that we could make a healing change by lowering biophoton emissions," explains Lynne. "We wanted to start with biophoton emissions because they are one of the most subtle of biological signals, and they are exquisitely sensitive. Any change—even a tiny change—can be readily picked up."

The duration of the experiment included six periods of 10 minutes of intention each, scattered at times unknown to the German laboratory staff across six hours, during which the biophoton and light-measuring equipment was turned on.

What did they find out? When the scientists graphed the light emissions, they discovered pronounced patterns of deviation from the normal symmetry of light distribution: The light patterns were profoundly altered during the exact periods when intention was sent. They also discovered a clear decrease in the amount of biophoton emissions among the targets during the meditation periods. Coincidence? The odds are incredibly remote. Some force had clearly affected the target subjects at these intervals, and there were no other new forces operating in the laboratory while the biophoton emissions were being measured. The only known additional force was the thought intention of the meditation subjects.

Certainly, this was an incredibly positive start. Since then, Lynne and the rest of the research group have continued to accumulate more evidence. Their experiments always follow standard scientific protocols for reducing or removing the chance of coincidence or random forces interfering with the results, including the use of control groups to compare test results and the blind method to remove observer bias, as well as the latest electronic gadgetry for measuring even the slightest variation in the material condition of the target objects.

As of April 2008, Lynne and her associates had run six separate experiments attempting to send intentions to make plants grow faster. In each instance, they consistently saw the target plants grow faster and taller than the controls, which were not sent intentions.

"We've had incredible evidence of a response every single time we've done it, whether it's been on the Internet or with a group that I've been speaking in front of. We've found that the seeds sent intention grow much higher than the controls, and we usually have three sets of controls."

The experiments have been run from as far away as Sydney, Australia, where intention senders send intentions to 30 seeds in Tucson, Arizona. Despite the thousands of miles of distance, they've seen results every time under very controlled conditions.

So what, you might say. What good is created by making some seeds grow? You have to appreciate the awesome scientific implications: *Thought is affecting matter.*

Lynne's research associate at the University of Arizona, Dr. Gary Schwartz, has done additional work in that area, testing purported energy healers in the United States and measuring the apparent power of their thoughts relative to "normal" people. When they ran seed experiments with a group of energy healers in South Carolina sending intentions, they found the plants that were sent intentions grew twice as high as the controls, more than they had ever seen previously.

For Lynne, the results produced by the energy healers demonstrated something very important: The power of intention is affected by practice and technique, and experience counts.

This finding inspired her to pursue a new avenue of research regarding the power of thought. She created a training program in effective techniques for improving the power of intention, based on the time-tested methods of different traditions around the world.

"It began to dawn on me from this evidence that the science shows we are actually senders and receivers of information every moment. When we use intention, we think of it as the big ask—the 'big thought'—our power thought. But actually, it's evident to me now that we are sending and receiving at every moment."

After looking at the science and talking with a wide variety of "intention masters" from many different philosophical and spiritual backgrounds, Lynne put together a set of basic practices and techniques to help people become better senders and receivers, inspired by the sages and practitioners whom she interviewed.

"Although they are people from completely different traditions, many of them have common techniques that all boil down to similar types of practices," Lynne explains. "For instance, all of them used some sort of focused mind state, so one of the things I work on is developing that high degree of focus."

Lynne calls her program "Powering up," and it draws on concentration techniques that would be recognizable to many meditation practitioners. She emphasizes that meditation isn't about "spacing out" or entering a sleepy dreamy state as some people believe. It's the opposite.

"The brain state that encourages a high degree of focus isn't a calming state, it's energized. You enter a zone, a kind of hyperspace. When I looked at the science, I actually found that the brains of Buddhist monks and master healers don't slow down. They speed up to a state that's higher than ordinary waking consciousness. And we can all work on these techniques to focus and energize our minds to a great degree."

In 2008, Lynne presented instruction in techniques such as "Powering up" to attendees at several "Living with Intention" workshops that she delivered across the United States to help people learn how to practise intention effectively on a day-to-day basis. Her workshops also addressed the power of group intention, where a collective body of people focusing with one intention can create even larger effects such as physical healings. Many people with chronic back pain and migraines reported healing effects. In one case, a woman who was nearly blind in one eye reported that 80 percent of her sight was restored.

In these workshop exercises, Lynne took her lead from the people in the online Intention Experiment community who had already been using group intention to heal each other. Using the guidelines from Lynne's website, readers have formed their own groups for practising intention, and they have reported healings that defy current Western medical understanding.

"There was one man, for instance, who had terrible burns on his hands," says Lynne. "He was in a gas explosion, and he was supposed to be in the hospital for months to get skin grafts. After receiving a powerful group intention, he was well enough to leave the hospital in six days. He didn't need skin grafts, and the doctors are considering him a medical miracle." This man's online Intention community had sent him a mere 10 minutes of healing intention each day; it certainly beats months in hospital with repeated visits to a medical surgeon. It also helps to highlight the power of intention in the healing process, which is similarly reflected in Bernie Siegel's work with terminal cancer patients.

Lynne certainly sees Bernie's work fitting well with the work that she and her group have been doing. She personally saw the power of hope at work when her mother-in-law had cancer a few years ago.

"She had end-stage breast cancer, and she was too late for all the ordinary stuff because she had nursed it privately. We brought her to a very good doctor who was interested in alternative approaches, like Dr. Siegel.

"The doctor looked at her breast, which was ravaged by the disease, and I listened to him when he examined her. He said, 'We can handle that.' And I knew at that moment she was going to get better because he was going to give her the best medicine that any doctor can give, which is hope. I've seen that in a lot of the research that I've looked at with the Intention Experiment. One after another, it's the thought that is the healer. Just look at the evidence for the placebo effect."

After the placebo effect and the healing power of hope, the implications and the possibilities for practising intention only get bigger. By teaching techniques such as "Powering up" and demonstrating the power of intention through large-scale experiments, Lynne hopes to help people feel they can have an impact in their community and ultimately the world at large. One of her concerns is that we have come to feel powerless amid dire and gloomy world events and circumstances, and she'd like to help people regain the confidence that they can have a positive effect on the well-being of the world.

"We're a really disempowered lot right now," says Lynne. "We feel very powerless with everything that's going on—recession looming, stress. I want us to move past that. I want to develop a way of doing this as a community."

So what's the key to successfully practising intention? The two keys are to be focused and communal. This moves us past the kind of incoherent, nonspecific messages that we usually broadcast to the world. Consequently, Lynne's guidelines for practising intention address the problems of incoherent thinking and instead generate intense mental focus.

The first step is to choose a place where you can practise intention on a regular basis. Research by Lynne and her colleagues has shown that using the same physical space adds power to the process. To create optimal chances of success, find a comfortable room or corner that you have consistent access to, and practise every day, even if it is just for five minutes.

But what does it mean to "practise"? The next steps form what Lynne calls "Powering up." There are essentially two parts to this process: The first is to enter a state of light meditation, and the second is to practise mindfulness to achieve "peak intensity."

To enter a state of light meditation, Lynne advocates a simple form of meditation that shares common features with many traditions. Distinct techniques are taught in different faiths and traditions, some far more complicated than others. The technique she recommends is informally called alpha meditation because your brain-wave activity slows from its normal waking state (dominated by beta waves) to the calmer level of alpha waves. Consistent with many forms of meditation, such as those taught by Buddhist teachers and other Eastern faiths, you practise basic rhythmic breathing to still your thoughts, and then you focus your mind on a steady "anchor" to keep your mind in this clear state. An anchor can be the sound and rhythm of your breath itself, a mantra, soft music with repetitive cycles or motifs, or a repetitive prayer. The outcome of this process is a deceleration of your brain-wave frequencies to the alpha state.

The next step is to practise mindfulness to achieve peak intensity in your conscious awareness. This is different from simply concentrating: Think of mindfulness as being calmly aware, watchful, attentive, and nonjudgmental to every appearance, sound, and sensation in your daily environment. This includes each sound of a passing car, or the sensation of a gentle breeze in your hair. It also includes paying attention to your feelings

Having stilled yourself in this watchful and aware state, you are now ready to create an empathetic connection. You do this by focusing your loving, compassionate thoughts on the person (or plant, or object). This works especially well with friends and people you know and love, but it isn't limited to them. As Lynne's studies have shown, complete strangers can and will benefit from your intention. She has found that if the focus of your intention is someone you don't know, then you can help the process by spending time with them (in person or online) or by exchanging a personal object or a photograph.

Next, from within your meditation, state the intention you wish to see fulfilled. Lynne recommends using the present tense, as though the intention has already been made reality. In her book *The Intention Experiment*, she gives this example for healing back pain: "My lower back and sacrum are free of all pain and now move easily and fluidly." She also recommends that you make your intentions as specific as possible, including the details of who, what, when, where, why, and how, almost as a news reporter would. The greater the level of detail, the stronger the effect of your intention.

You then use these details to form a visualization of the final result of your intention. That is, you create a mental image or feeling of your intention when it is fulfilled. If you are someone who is naturally inclined toward mental imagery and your visual senses, you might find it easier to form an actual picture in your mind. However, if you are someone who is less visually oriented and more tactile, you can manifest a feeling or sensation in your body of how it *feels* to have this intention fulfilled. To strengthen your ability in this area, you can practise your visualization process by meditating and then gently recreating in your mind all of the sensory details of a recent happy experience, such as listening to music, being with a loved one, or enjoying good food or drink.

When you send your intention, you need to believe that the process works. If you state your intentions while secretly believing that the process is mere wishful thinking and not real, then you drain the power from your intentions. This much should be obvious, given that we are talking about the power of thought: You can't harbor two beliefs that work at opposite purposes to one another. Belief is part of the bedrock of your visualization process. Without it, the intention lacks backbone and resolve.

You also have to "step aside" after you send your intentions. You need to recognize that the power of intention works through a larger field of energy consciousness in the universe, not from you in the individual sense *per se*. You are simply directing energy that is already in motion in the quantum soup around us, and applying it to a specific target and purpose.

Finally, you may wish to look at sending your intentions at times of optimal solar activity. The surface of the sun produces solar activity in the form of sunspots and solar flares that vary in size and frequency over days, weeks, and months, and these events in turn have an effect on the earth's geomagnetic field (GMF). Intense solar activity causes geomagnetic storms in space that cause fluctuations in the GMF, which in turn affects everything from satellite and aircraft communications to our own central nervous system and brain waves. Lynne says there is evidence that acts of psychokinesis, such as sending thought intentions, work better during active solar periods when the GMF is stormy. (By contrast, when the GMF is calm, intention may be less effective, but telepathy and extrasensory perception improve.) You can actually check the solar weather forecast by visiting the website of the U.S. National Oceanic and Atmospheric Administration and consulting the Space Weather Prediction Center forecast (see http://www.swpc.noaa.gov). According to Lynne, your intentions will receive the biggest boost in power when you time them to coincide with GMF activity that registers high in the K-index, a scale used to measure geomagnetic turbulence. The K-index ranges from 1 to 9, and Lynne suggests that you send your intentions on days when the K-index is 5 or more if you want to maximize the effect of your effort.

"But probably the most important thing is developing techniques of a certain emotional state," says Lynne. "It's about changing your brain to become a better perceiver of information *and* a better sender, perceiving the world slightly differently."

Using intention has many similarities to discussions of the Law of Attraction in that both recommend that you visualize your desired end result in order to manifest it. However, there are subtle distinctions that are important. For instance, in contrast to proponents of the Law of Attraction, Lynne feels cautious about making sweeping generalizations as to how we can reshape every aspect of our lives, such as personal wealth and relationships.

"What we're really looking at is affecting matter, not necessarily affecting all life events," she explains. "I think *The Secret* was very good because it introduced so many people to these ideas in a very, very simple way. The question is really how far can we go?"

For her part, Lynne is more interested in what group intention can do for larger numbers of people on a larger geographical scale. For instance, in 2008, Lynne and the group ran intention experiments in purifying water samples and manifesting peace in the strife-torn northern portion of Sri Lanka. If the group can demonstrate the power of intention at this scale (data from these experiments were still being analyzed at the time of this writing), then Lynne believes we can feel empowered as individuals and begin to understand that our collective thoughts are capable of changing the world. The implications and possibilities are endless, and they begin with learning new habits to make the most of our intentions.

"I think for people to get to the next stage, and to really make it effective, we are going to have to open ourselves to some very, very unusual new things. We're brought up with an old scientific story. We're brought up with a sense of our own separation at every moment, and yet the new science shows us we're actually part of a unity. We're part of one great big energy field, and we can influence the world around us. We are a dynamic power for good. We have to begin to perceive this with new eyes. We have to learn new ways of being."

Considering the existing findings of the Intention Experiment in making plants grow and in healing people, I think we can already be confident in our ability to shape this world. The next step is to practise focusing and aiming this ability consciously, sending the greatest good to where it is most needed. This kind of intentionality may also play a role in our personal relationships. As we will see in our next chapter, science has made similar breakthroughs in our understanding of how mental "maps" shape much of our partnering behavior.

FALLING IN LOVE

chapter 6

with HELEN FISHER

Dr. Helen Fisher is a leading expert in the science of what makes us love. Currently research professor at the Center for Human Evolutionary Studies in the Department of Anthropology, Rutgers University, she has been studying and writing about the evolution of human sex, love, and marriage for more than 25 years.

"Never give up on Cupid: The brain circuit for romantic love is fickle and mysterious, and it can be triggered at any time."

She is the author of four books: *Why We Love: The Nature and Chemistry of Romantic Love; The First Sex: The Natural Talents of Women and How They Are Changing the World; Anatomy of Love: The Natural History of Monogamy, Adultery, and Divorce;* and *The Sex Contract: The Evolution of Human Behavior.*

Living joyfully is a challenge put to us not only as individuals, but one that extends to the joy that we can create with others through our relationships. Loving human relationships are key avenues for reaching our full, healthy expression as human beings, forming an essential element in the process of becoming healthy as a whole. They provide exhilarating possibilities for expressing ourselves spiritually, mentally, and physically as we move toward greater self-knowledge and awareness. While you will learn a great deal about the spiritual benefits of human relationships throughout the book, in this chapter Dr. Helen Fisher will introduce you to the latest science concerning mating, dating, and falling in love.

As a biological anthropologist and expert in the science of human attraction, Dr. Fisher's insights will surprise you. For example, despite the widespread belief that the institution of marriage is in decline, Helen says it has actually grown stronger in the last 20 years, and it is certainly much stronger than it was in centuries past.

"For centuries people thought your devotion to kin and to God were more important than your devotion to a spouse. Historians say that strong marital commitments only became the foundation stone of society in the twentieth century. With the rise of the isolated nuclear family, people began to expect more from their marriages, including deep intimacy and companionship. In fact, the number of people who have important conversations *only* with a spouse doubled between 1985 and 2004, from 5 percent to almost 10 percent. This reflects how we work harder today on our partnerships than we did at any time in Western history."

What about the statistics that indicate the marriage rate has been falling in the United States? This is a good example of how statistics don't tell the whole story.

"People today are concerned that the marriage rate is falling, but I don't think this is something to worry about. Ninety percent of Americans will marry by middle age—they're just doing it later. Today the marriage rate is falling largely because the *remarriage* rate is falling, and the remarriage rate is falling because the divorce rate is falling. In fact, the divorce rate in America is down to 43 percent—down from almost 50 percent in the early 1980s, so if you don't get divorced, you're not going to get remarried."

People are still getting married, but they are simply waiting longer to do it, and there are fewer remarriages because there are actually fewer divorces. When you view these factors together, it's clear that love and marriage remain strong forces in our society.

Still, statistics aren't half as interesting as understanding the actual physical, emotional, and psychological mechanics of love. Helen has always wanted to know precisely how love functions within us, so in one of her studies, she hooked up love-struck individuals to MRI machines to see what happens in their brains. Using the MRI data, she looked at which neural networks are activated when people feel romantic love, as distinct from passion or attachment.

"The most active brain regions in romantic love are the ventral tegmental area, a small factory near the base of the brain that produces dopamine and sends it to many brain regions, and the caudate nucleus, a brain area the size of a medium-sized shrimp on either side of the head. Both the VTA and caudate are part of a major circuit, the reward system, the system associated with focused attention, motivation, goal-oriented behaviors, craving, and the rush of intense romantic love."

Helen's 2004 book *Why We Love* describes some of the research findings. She talks about romantic love around the world and how it was not invented by the troubadours, and she also goes into the poetry, myths, legends, songs, and love magic that indicate that everywhere people love. The research suggests we have evolved three distinctly different brain systems for mating and reproduction: one being the sex drive, the second being romantic love, and the third being attachment, or that sense of common security you often feel with a long-term partner. Sentiments of attachment are less urgent or intense than romantic love, and the lustful physical urge of the sex drive is, of course, distinct from both of them.

"Some people confuse romantic love with the sex drive. Actually, these are *very* different networks in the brain with very different feelings. The sex drive is the craving for sexual gratification—W.H. Auden called it an intolerable neural itch—and you can feel the sex drive for a range of partners.

"Romantic love is very different. Foremost, it is focused on just *one* person and, although you would *like* to have sex with him or her, even more important, you want them to call and to write and to ask you out, and to create emotional union with you. So sex and romantic love are different feelings, but in a good relationship, of course, most people want both."

Best value in a relationship is having "intercourse" of both kinds. Healthy sex is a natural expression of our physical natures, and it can even be good exercise. At the same time, the type of insightful communication and common understanding that comes from a deeper romantic connection creates a sense of mutual security and validation of who we are, satisfying our innate drive toward increased self-awareness and self-actualization.

This leads to the next question: What kind of person lights up those parts of our brain that make us lust and love? To answer this question, Helen has studied how our blend of genetics and social conditioning affects what we look for in a romantic partner. As she puts it, we all carry a kind of internal checklist or template that we use to assess potential partners—a "love map." If we can understand our love maps and how they are created, we can understand what each of us may be seeking in a romantic partner and how we're likely to go about winning them.

It has long been the stuff of high romance to think that each of us has only one ideal partner waiting for us somewhere out there in the world, and today this belief persists with people who talk about finding their perfect soul mate. But it may be a different kind of predestination that defines our partnering habits, a destiny that is determined largely by our biology and psychology.

Research shows that we are not limited to only one potential partner or soul mate. Our checklist for a partner generally allows for a good number of potential romantic candidates, though we may be limited in our shopping selection by geography and other factors. Helen has acquired additional insight into identifying those factors through her work as chief scientific advisor to Chemistry.com, the Internet dating site geared to people seeking partners for long-term relationships. By looking at aggregate data from the traffic on the site, she has been able to formulate a few hypotheses on what makes people choose one person over another and succumb to love.

"I think we have a list of traits that we're looking for in a mate, or what I call your love map. When the timing is right, any number of people who fit within this template can trigger that brain circuit for romantic passion, and you can fall head over heels in love."

When is the timing "right?" It's almost impossible to predict. Our partnering behavior is influenced by countless variables that are always changing in value. For example, we have hormonal levels that fluctuate according to factors such as age and diet. Then there are simple situational factors that determine who we're likely to meet as prospective partners, such as where we live, what we do for work, and how socially active we are. It creates a complex array of possibilities in timing that we don't have a lot of control over.

Much of your love map is determined by your social background, ethnicity, culture, and even level of income and education. Each of us has a different map, so it's very difficult to predict where and when you'll become enamored. Then there are genetic factors and even geographical considerations—we tend to fall in love with the people who are simply around us!

"Psychologists know that we tend to gravitate to people who have the same ethnic background, same socio-economic background, same religious values, same general level of intelligence, same general level of good looks, and these days the same general level of education, but this is all they know.

They know that your childhood plays a role, but they really haven't quantified that."

The dearth of more specific indicators for what makes us fall in love was a big motivator for Helen to conduct much of her own research. Especially in her work with Chemistry. com, she realized that she needed a better set of criteria for predicting which types of people would make successful partnerships.

"When you give really good personality questionnaires to people who have been married for 20 years, you find no patterns at all, other than what I've just said. For example, in terms of personality, extroverts don't necessarily gravitate to extroverts; people who are thrill-seekers don't necessarily gravitate to other thrill-seekers, etc. So reading all of this data, I realized I need to know a little bit more about what people are looking for if I'm going to help match them."

Helen's research took her deeper into the realm of human genetics and literally the physical chemistry of what makes us love. She looked at the genetic component of personality and considered different biological types, and she began to form a hypothesis of what biological variables create the love spark.

"Fifty percent of personality is called temperament, and this is directed by your DNA," says Helen. "For example, the degree to which you are curious has a genetic component. The degree to which you are cautious, and the degree to which you trust—these have a genetic component. Cautiousness is linked with specific genes in the serotonin system, while trust is linked with oxytocin."

The genetic variations create different biological types, and the behavior of these types reflects their biology. She calls the type who expresses many genes in the serotonin system the "Builder."

"These people are calm, social, cautious, managerial, literal, detail-oriented, conventional, and often religious. Colin Powel and Sarah Palin are examples."

She calls a person who expresses a lot of oxytocin and estrogen the "Negotiator."

"These people see the big picture. They are imaginative, intuitive, verbally skilled, have good people skills, and are compassionate. Bill Clinton is a good example."

These genetic factors and the biological types explain why you might be attracted to only some of the individuals who otherwise meet all of your "love map" criteria.

"Within a large pool of people with whom we share similar education, intelligence, religious values, etc., we're not attracted to everybody. We're only attracted to some of them. My hypothesis is that we gravitate to people who are somewhat chemically and genetically different from us because for millions of years, it would have been adaptive to pool your DNA with somebody who was somewhat different, so you could create more genetic variety in your babies and come to the job of parenting with a wider array of parenting skills."

Those who sought some degree of biological novelty in their mating tended to be more successful reproductively. They reproduced and thrived, and they passed on to their children the predisposition to seek a degree of variety in their partners. Consequently, we have these brain mechanisms today that when we walk into a room and everyone's from our background, and everyone shares our religious values and so forth, we tend to unconsciously gravitate to people who are somewhat chemically different from us.

To some degree we also form partnerships on the basis of *exchange theory*. Basically, an element of attraction is whether or not our prospective partners can give us what we need in exchange for what they need. The classic example is the rich elderly man marrying the young beautiful woman, but the exchange can be anything, and it's not always so evident. Sometimes our needs are determined by what we lack. If we're broke, we tend to be attracted to people who have a job, or if we're very skilled in math, we might be attracted to a poet to complement our analytical personality. We're also attracted to people who provide us with the opportunity to play certain roles. We might like the idea of being the "husband of a university president" or the "wife of a corporate executive." Conversely, we may decide we're not interested in being the "wife of a traveling salesman" or the "husband of a navy diesel engineer." The bottom line is that both partners have to think that there's a fair exchange being made, and when they do, they tend to be happier in the partnership.

If exchange theory disturbs your romantic view of love, keep in mind that exchange is only one of many factors that might influence your selection of a partner—love is still more than simple barter and trade. For example, love can be its own reason. Other research has found that men and women simply tend to fall in love with someone who's in love with them.

"In a sample of several hundred Americans and Israelis, 47 percent of women and 35 percent of men said that knowing that their suitor was *crazy* about them played an important role in turning feelings of passion, into a trip to the altar. As the poet Theodore Roethke said, 'Love begets love.' To *get* love, you often have to *give* it."

Is this self-interested love? In a manner of speaking, yes, but it's not necessarily "bad" or even unusual. As Helen will tell you, almost all behavior has some advantages to the self; otherwise it wouldn't have evolved. Remember, our romantic partnerships are as much about discovering ourselves as they are about coming to understand and appreciate the person we give flowers to on Valentine's Day. Someone who loves us is helping us to feel validated as a human being, and validation gives us motivation to continue living, learning, and growing. That's healthy. Without some degree of validation, we don't feel at ease in the world, and our self-doubts can lead to crippling depression, so we shouldn't judge anyone too harshly for falling in love with someone because the other person loves him or her.

The question is whether or not it's enough for you to actually fall in love at that point. With all of the different factors and elements of timing involved, it's not a given. There still has to be some sort of romantic chemistry. Sometimes chemistry takes a while to develop, so we may need to be patient when we're dating someone. Some of us fall in love very quickly, but for others, it may take months or even years.

Helen recounts a touching story about a couple who took a while to realize what they had.

"I know one man who courted a woman for almost four years. Then one day during a lovely stroll through Central Park in New York, after they'd had an elegant lunch together and some heady and some humorous conversation, she fell madly in love with him. And she's still in love with him nine years later, so I would never give up on Cupid. The brain circuit for romantic love is fickle and mysterious, and it can be triggered at any time."

Some people may need time to develop feelings of trust before they enter into romance, or they might simply need time to develop an appreciation for what you offer as a person and a prospective partner. Part of this reflects how our romantic needs can sometimes change with time.

The research shows that the fundamental *traits* we're looking for in a mate do not change, but our *priorities* may change as we travel through life. In high school we might be looking for a football star or somebody in a rock band, but as we mature, we begin to look for someone who will help us raise a family, go hiking in the mountains, or enjoy sailing. However, while our larger priorities might change, the basic aspects of our "love map"—our unconscious list of traits that we're looking for in a partner—do *not* change. If you were drawn to people who were curious, religious, or amusing when you were young, you will still gravitate toward these traits in a partner even in your nineties.

And according to Helen, everyone does fall in love. Everywhere in the world, almost everyone falls prey to love's spell, but it might take years or even decades for some people to meet the special person who matches their love map criteria. Timing plays a huge role in who we meet—where, when, and in what state of receptivity to romance.

"I've met two people actually—one man and one woman—who had never felt that exhilaration, craving, or excessive thinking of romantic love until their mid-fifties," recounts Helen. "Both were married, both fell in love with somebody else, and both were eventually very faithful to their spouses. But both had a hard time for a few years, and both told me the same thing: They said that they finally understood plays like *Romeo and Juliet*."

Just about everybody falls in love at some point in their lives, so you should never give up. Romantic love is a basic brain circuit that can be triggered at any time, so it *will* happen to you. You might feel this kind of passion rarely or only once in your lifetime, or you might find that you're the type who falls in love on a regular basis. Scientists don't yet know why some people are more prone to romantic love than others, but Helen suspects that it probably has something to do with the activity of dopamine in the brain, the neurotransmitter that produces romantic passion.

"It's just part of human variation. Some people are more sexual, some are more daring, some are more curious, some are more enthusiastic. People vary in lots of ways, due both to their biology and their experiences. The people I know who fall in love all the time learn to ignore it. They don't act on it because they want to preserve the relationship that they've got with their long-term partner."

But, of course, the million-dollar question is: How can you tell if someone is in love with you?

"Sometimes it's difficult, particularly if they're very good at hiding their feelings," says Helen. "But normally when someone's in love, they call, they write, they make an enormous effort to see you again and again, and when they do see you, they're likely to ask you all sorts of questions about yourself and remember the answers. They will also be full of energy, their eyes will sparkle, and they will smile and laugh easily.

"Another giveaway is when they begin to act awkward around you. It's called the sweaty palm syndrome because they'll sweat, they'll shake, they'll stammer—all signs of this intense chemical reaction. If someone begins to act a little bit goofy or too intense, they're probably in love with you."

When you and that special someone find each other, how can you keep the relationship happy and vital? After all, if you're someone who is fortunate enough to have bonded with a loving partner, you probably want to keep the relationship intact. Helen has a few strategies to offer you, though strictly from the viewpoint of an anthropologist. She likes to make it clear that she is *not* a relationship counselor!

"Basically you want to sustain three distinctly different brain networks: the sex drive, romantic love, and feelings of deep attachment. To trigger the sex drive, have sex. Sex stimulates testosterone and it can jump-start your desire for more sex, as well as bring intimacy. To sustain romantic love, do novel things together. Novelty drives up dopamine in the brain and can sustain feelings of romantic passion. And to trigger attachment, hold hands, walk arm-in-arm, or touch in some other way. Touching can trigger the brain's oxytocin, giving you feelings of trust and union with a sweetheart."

Renewing the novelty of your relationship is something you can achieve, at least in part, by making time for dates with your partner. Too many people allow themselves to grow complacent in their relationship—whether it's due to the pressures of raising children, working long hours, or simply lack of initiative—and they forget to do the fun and novel things as a couple that would help to nourish their love. You need to recognize the *relationship* as an entity in its own right, and do things to keep it healthy.

"I think there are three people in a relationship: You, your partner, and the relationship. The relationship needs attention too, so if you want to keep your partnership strong, make regular dates with your spouse. Every couple of weeks, go out and do some of the things that you used to do when you were courting—dress up, flirt, go somewhere new, have an adventure."

Because novelty stimulates dopamine in the brain, your new dating adventures will help to stimulate the neural networks that make you feel passionate. Dopamine can also trigger testosterone, which is the hormonal driver for physical lust. Helen also offers this advice: Laugh with your lover. To North Americans, laughter is happiness, and happiness is a great bonding agent between two people!

If you are looking at your current romance, or if you're searching for a romantic partner, consider some of the points that Helen raises. First of all, give some thought to what constitutes your "love map," the various traits and qualities that you are seeking in an ideal lover. Some of these may be obvious to you, and others less so, but it will be helpful for you understand what you value in your relationship. You might find that there are areas of your current partnership that you want to improve, or if you are looking for a new partner, you will find it useful to know what you're looking for as it will help you to determine how and where you might meet these types of partners. Remember that some of the strongest determinants of who you partner with are based on simple traits: similar income, level of education, similar level of good looks, ethnicity, and cultural background. However, the rest of your love formula gets tricky because it relies to a great extent on the timing of who you meet and when, as well as your DNA and the chemistry of oxytocin, estrogen, testosterone, and serotonin in your system. In that sense, you will always have to leave some of your romancing to chance.

When you do find that special someone, remember to continue nourishing your relationship. Do novel things, laugh a lot, and you'll be able to enjoy all three dimensions of love with your partner for the long term—rewarding sex, meaningful attachment, and intriguing romance. If you have all of these qualities working in your partnership, you will be well on your way to finding happiness and health in your life.

SECTION 2

We have looked at the health of our mind and some of the powerful transformations that can happen when we work on our mental perceptions and intentions. The next step is to consider the health of your body, the physical vehicle that will enable your mind and spirit to reach their full potential. If we wish to live full lives as parents and lovers, or develop the greatest capacities of our mind through study, or seek spiritual insight through contemplative work such as meditation, a healthy physical vehicle will enhance all of these activities.

Your physical health is nurtured through a few basic practices: good diet, appropriate supplementation, and regular exercise suitable to your age. In the next four chapters, we will closely examine the latest findings in exercise, fighting fat, and supplementing according to your needs using the best in proven plant remedies and the latest in natural supplements.

Of course, what and how you eat are also important factors in your physical health, and you should always pursue good dietary planning to ensure optimal nutrition. However, a long discussion of diet is beyond the scope of this book. There are hundreds, if not thousands, of diet books available to help you get your nutrition in order. Instead, in our next chapters, we will delve a little more

HEALTH
OF BODY

deeply into key topics in physical health that might be less familiar to most people.

Two of these involve new research into the importance of exercise and fighting weight gain—a growing health issue now facing the developed world in particular—and another focuses on how you can boost your health with natural nutritional supplements and plant remedies, avoiding the often serious side effects and risks of pharmaceutical medicines and synthetic products.

As with mental and spiritual practices, it's possible to over-indulge ourselves and become preoccupied exclusively with regimens and programs dedicated to physical health and fitness. I encourage you to pursue a holistic approach where you develop your physical wellness in balance with your mental and spiritual needs. Conversely, if you already tend to emphasize mental and spiritual activity in your life, then you may need to make an extra effort to pay attention to your physical needs. In short, we need to practise diligence in eating right, supplementing correctly, and exercising regularly to ensure that our bodies are the optimized vehicles we would like them to be, all while coordinating our efforts with the activity of our mental, emotional, and spiritual lives. The following chapters will introduce you to the latest insights in this area.

FIT TO LIVE

chapter 7

with DR. PAMELA PEEKE

Dr. Pamela Peeke is one of America's leading educators and researchers in holistic health, nutrition, and fitness. She is an assistant professor of medicine at the University of Maryland, the Pew Foundation scholar in nutrition and metabolism, the chief medical

This is about more than just trying to fit into a swimsuit or a pair of pants . . . healthy habits allow us to increase our joy of living.

correspondent for Discovery Health TV, a member of Oprah Winfrey's medical expert panel, and the host of Discovery TV's "Could You Survive . . . Are You Fit to Live?" She is also author of multiple national best-selling books, including the *New York Times* best-seller, *Body for Life for Women*.

There are several key factors to maintaining physical health and vitality. Some are obvious, like the need to keep our weight in a suitable range for our age and thereby reduce our risk factors for a number of diseases. Others are less obvious, such as the need to reduce our stress levels so we can maintain healthy immune systems and slow our aging process. We need to adopt a variety of healthy practices regarding diet, exercise, and attitude to achieve these aims, which might seem a daunting task for many of us, but here's the good news: It's possible to break the larger goal of physical wellness into practical, manageable habits to achieve our physical fitness priorities, and Dr. Pamela Peeke is one of the people who can tell us how.

Dr. Pamela Peeke is one of America's leading educators and researchers in holistic health, nutrition, and fitness. In addition to writing about fitness and developing exercise programs, she's an avid athlete and fitness enthusiast herself, and her taut physique and physical exuberance have earned her the epithet "The doc who walks the talk." She is a vocal advocate of combating fat and the stresses of modern living through balanced exercise and diet, especially in the area of women's health and weight loss, and she provides an even larger set of wellness principles to help you stay healthy in all areas of your life—physically, mentally, financially, and environmentally.

Pam's passion for physical fitness began with her early research into obesity and the negative health effects of being 'even moderately overweight. In her book *Fight Fat after Forty*, Pam looks at the connections between stress and fat, reflecting on much of her research with the National Institutes of Health. She presents a new world of concern about the dangers of carrying a spare tire around your waist, and she has started a buzz about what she calls "toxic fat," an excess of intra-abdominal fat deep inside the midriff that can interact with your insulin, glucose, and liver to cause significant health issues.

In a nutshell, stress tends to increase the visceral fat in your intra-abdominal area, and as a result, your risk for heart disease, diabetes, and cancer increases. The research shows that you can have very little fat on your hips or thighs and look relatively trim, but an excess of deep belly fat could still be increasing your risk factors for these diseases. The stress connection is clear.

Pam's book was the first to explain the science of fat in laypeople's terms.

"I concentrated on people over the age of 40 because that's when you begin to see body fat on the rise in just about everyone. But it isn't only about the quantity of fat in your body; it is also about the quality."

As Pam points out, it's not just about how much fat you have. We can all recognize people who are obviously overweight or obese, but Pam reveals something startling that is much less apparent to the eye: It's possible for you to have an overall body weight that fits your correct body mass index (BMI) according to your height and weight, yet still be on the brink of ill health due to having body fat in the *wrong* place—around your waist.

"I call it toxic fat. Everyone has fat deep in their belly. You have to for a multitude of reasons. It helps regulate your core body temperature; it buffers your organs; it's a great little repository of extra fat fuel, but the problem is when you have too much of a good thing.

"When we have *too much* fat deep in the belly, we all run into huge problems: heart disease, diabetes, and cancer. . . . It is really important for people today, especially people over 40, to change their mindset about fat. We have heard the messages about staying slim for decades, but now we have to refine our understanding. It's no longer how fat you are—*it's where the fat is at.* You can be a completely absolutely normal body weight, and still have too great a girth."

When we look at our waistlines and take into account this new understanding of toxic fat, the question on everyone's mind is: How much is too much? Pam's guidelines are effective and very simple to follow. Pull out a tape measure and wrap it around your waist at belly-button level. For women, health risks increase when waist circumference exceeds 35 inches; for men, 40 inches is the upper limit. The newest evidence shows that your girth is a far more effective predictor of health or ill health than any of the older tools, including your overall weight and your BMI, so forget about whether or not you "appear" to be fit. Take a close look at the circumference around your belly button and see how it compares to the 35/40 rule.

Many of us will find that we are close to or over this maximum. This means that chances are high that we are carrying the toxic fat that Pam talks about, especially if we are over 40 years of age when there's a tendency to acquire more of it. There are a number of reasons why our abdominal fat in particular begins to accumulate at that time. The first reason is lifestyle.

"The reality is that toxic fat is caused by poor lifestyle habits. If you overeat and you're not exercising, or not getting a decent level of physical activity, you will be storing more and more fat, and some of it is going to go straight to the problem area—you're going to end up storing it deep in your belly.

"Another contributing factor is declining sex hormones in both men and women. Declining testosterone and estrogen levels are linked to fat storage in our bodies. Men's testosterone will drop at the rate of roughly 5–8 percent per decade starting at the age of 40. For women, you're going through a slow but sure estrogen *withdrawal*, and this is when that 'meno-pot' starts showing up, but that's just *outside* the abdominal muscle wall. Inside, if our lifestyle habits are not optimal, it becomes much easier for women to store toxic fat right where we least want it."

The third main cause is chronic stress, a major feature of our modern lives in the developed world. Chronic stress is different from having a tough day or being in an argument; it is an ongoing physical state wherein your stress hormones, particularly adrenaline and cortisol, are constantly elevated. Cortisol, in particular, stimulates fat cells in the abdomen to increase in size. It encourages fat storage. It has also been shown to slow metabolism, increase food cravings, and deregulate your blood sugar balance. As Pam says, it's funny how tuna on a bed of greens never quite does it when you're stressed out. When your levels of cortisol are chronically elevated, your immune system begins to erode and you age faster. You tend to get colds and flu more often, and you increase your risk of developing serious long-term illnesses such as cancer and heart disease. Clearly, we want to discover ways to decrease stress and keep our cortisol levels in check!

In her most recent book *Fit to Live*, Pam presents a five-point plan for promoting physical fitness and basic wellness so we can survive, thrive, and be "lean, strong, and fearless for life." The three physical components of her plan are mind, mouth, and muscle. In addition to these, she offers two more M's for a complete, integrative approach to wellness: money and macrocosm.

It's no shocker to think that we need to maintain ourselves with good basic nutrition (mouth), exercise (muscle), and right attitudes and mental well-being (mind). But we also need to be aware of how "healthy" we are financially (money) and whether or not we are living in balance with the environment around us (macrocosm). If either of these two latter factors is mismanaged, they have the potential to contribute more stress and toxicity to our lives and upset the apple cart of everything we do with mouth, muscle, and mind, and then we're just feeding the cycle that leads back to toxic fat and disease.

"When you're not paying attention to mind, mouth, muscle, money, and macrocosm, in each one of those cases you'll end up self-destructively overeating, not exercising, or doing other things that are self-destructive. It ends up being reflected, believe it or not, in your girth."

You can't live a full life if you're sickly, stressed, and battling your weight. Even if you're not outright ill, carrying extra weight will seriously limit your ability to play with your children or grandchildren, hike outdoors, and take part in the many other activities that actually help to decrease stress and increase your enjoyment of life. This is about more than just trying to fit into a swimsuit, a dress, or a pair of pants. Again, we see how healthy habits allow us to increase our joy of living, and joy is the basic building block of human health. So, how can you take this knowledge and use it to improve your physical well-being?

For starters, address your muscle needs by getting started on a regular program of exercise that suits your interests and works where you live. Maybe you're not interested in playing shinny hockey, touch football, or golf, but you might enjoy walking, hiking, or swimming. Get a calendar of programs at your local recreational center, and talk to friends or workmates who might be interested in working together on a fitness program.

Educate yourself on good nutrition so you have the needs of your mouth met. There are many good books, but if reading about glycemic indexes, body mass indexes, and calories makes your head spin, this might not be a good route for you. Do what works. We know that our bodies have innate wisdom, but we also know it can be difficult to clear away the chatter in order to hear and understand the messages we are receiving. One of the best ways to practise this important skill is to listen closely to the signals you receive during and after eating different foods—and respond to them! As you get better at listening to your body's physical responses to what you eat, you will find that your new listening skills can be fine-tuned to receive ever more subtle cues that will guide you in your mental and spiritual work.

To address the concerns of the mind, take an inventory of the elements in your life that contribute to your stress levels, and look at your mental attitudes affecting wellness and weight.

Are you ready to choose something better for yourself? It all starts with you deciding to change your habits. Sometimes we don't get out of the starting blocks on a new diet or exercise regimen simply because we haven't made a determined choice, or we haven't removed simple environmental stresses or avoided situations that are toxic to us.

The money element plays a big role in managing stress. Reduce additional financial stressors in your life by being realistic about your current situation, and taking empowered steps to relieve yourself of significant money issues that are keeping you awake at night. Sound impossible? Keep in mind that countless studies have shown that stress about finances is linked to your *perception* of your current situation. You don't need to be rich or live an extravagant lifestyle to be happy. It is about learning to recognize the joy that comes from living simply, with gratitude, and within your means.

Finally, look at getting out and reconnecting with the natural world of the macrocosm around you. As Pam points out, far too many of us suffer from *nature deficiency*. We seldom get outside the mall and away from the asphalt, concrete, glass, and steel of our manufactured environments, and we have lost something of ourselves through our subsequent disconnect with nature. It's funny how the simple joy that comes from being in nature—such as contemplating a stream, walking in a forest, or lying in a meadow—can reduce much of our anxiety and worry about our work, our family, and other stressors.

So build a program for yourself, and draw on whatever family, friends, professionals, videos, CDs, library books, and other resources you need to make it happen. Get determined to get fit with all aspects of mind, mouth, muscle, money, and macrocosm. As you get these elements working together in a healthy direction, you'll find renewed joy and energy, and you'll be pleased to discover that you're physically, mentally, and spiritually stronger to enjoy the gift of this life, as well as rebound better when it deals you a wild card.

With regard to your muscles and body composition, we are going to get you started right now. In our next chapter, Sean Foy will show you how to incorporate a highly effective exercise program into your daily routine, even when you're immersed in a weekly whirl of family and career obligations.

WORKING OUT WITH 4-3-2-1
chapter 8

with SEAN FOY

Sean Foy is president and founder of Personal Wellness Corporation, a California-based firm that provides health and fitness consulting, educational seminars, and personal fitness training to corporations, hospitals, universities, and private clients. His firm also works with The Center for Optimal Health in Buena Park, California, to deliver fitness programming to people across the United

> *"My favorite results are the mental, spiritual, and relational aspects of becoming fit . . . motion affects emotion."*

States and internationally. He's also a coauthor with Dr. William Sears of the 2003 book, *LEAN Kids*, which presents parents with a complete program for addressing the optimal lifestyle, exercise, and nutrition for children ages six to 12. Sean has a new book coming out soon and we'll take a sneak peak at some of its highlights in this chapter.

Thanks to Dr. Pamela Peeke, we now understand that exercise is about more than just looking good, and that it's actually critical to avoiding toxic fat so we can live well and age gracefully. Now we're ready to learn how to do it. To keep the pounds off and maintain the physical abilities that we need to live a full life, we need an exercise regimen that addresses all of the components considered essential to comprehensive physical wellness: cardiovascular health, overall muscle strength and tone, core strength, and flexibility. At the same time, we also need a program that fits into our frantic daily and weekly schedules. With today's modern lifestyles, we're all busy all the time. We have to be able to follow our fitness plan while working, raising kids, taking care of aging parents, traveling, getting to appointments, running errands, and meeting all the other tasks and demands that constitute our often-hurried lives.

Fitness expert Sean Foy, the president and founder of California-based Personal Wellness Corporation, has designed an extremely effective exercise program that fits into anyone's busy schedule and still addresses all four essential physical capacities. As Sean teaches, you *can* get your fitness dose when you need it, even while building your career and caring for your family.

When I participated in the Orange County Marathon in early 2008, I had the opportunity to meet with Sean in Buena Park, and he took me on a guided tour of the Center for Optimal Health. The Center now conducts leading-edge health assessments to provide clients with a picture of their health at that moment and then, using these diagnostics, each client is able to identify weaknesses in his or her diet or exercise routines and make improvements. The Center does everything from blood chemistry analysis to comprehensive health and fitness testing, providing education on exactly what clients need to improve or maximize their health.

"It's been eight years since we've been working with the Center," says Sean. "People from all over the world have come through, and what we're seeing is dramatic. We see individuals losing weight, improving their body composition, blood cholesterol and blood pressure, and decreasing their major risk factors significantly. We provide them with the testing and also the education they need, and then we coach them through this process of change. What's fascinating and what's been exciting for us is hearing feedback from people about their barriers to staying fit, particularly when it comes to exercise."

Sean and his team have spent time developing a personal fitness program that addresses those barriers in a truly twenty-first-century way. At a time when people are squeezed for time between work and home schedules, Sean has put together a super-fast personal workout that addresses all of the main elements of a comprehensive exercise program in just 10 minutes a day, and it's producing big results.

"My program is called the 10-Minute Total Body Makeover," says Sean. "It is designed to help people improve their health and fitness with just 10 minutes of exercise a day. We've been absolutely overwhelmed by the response, not only physically but also psychologically."

Sean's program is based on a new approach to exercising that he invented. It's called 4-3-2-1 Fitness, and it's designed to help people become fit at what Sean calls "the speed of life." Each mini-workout routine can be done in just 10 minutes, and the workouts are so flexible they can be performed at home, at the office, outdoors, on the road, or at the gym.

"Over the years, I found that when I told people the basic exercise recommendations—three to five days a week of aerobic activity, plus a minimum of two to three days of resistance training, and don't forget regular stretching—most people would look at me and say, 'You've got to be kidding me—there's no way that I'm going to have the time to do all of that.' I realized that the greatest barrier for most people, especially in the U.S., is our busy schedules. I began testing a comprehensive fitness program that could be boiled down into a 10-minute circuit."

Following this 10-minute workout, you can address every essential fitness component to ensure you are strong, lean, flexible, and fit. Sean's program addresses every aspect of your physical health, including a cardiovascular workout, resistance training, core exercises, and deep breathing and stretching. Let's take a look at what this revolutionary program requires, and learn how to get started right away:

Four minutes of high-energy aerobic training, or HEAT: This is the cardiovascular component. Periods of high-intensity exercise are alternated with periods of recovery. This is a highly effective fitness technique known as interval training.

Three minutes of compound resistance exercises and thermic effect, or CREATE: This component of the workout is composed of three separate weight-training exercises that strengthen muscles and boost metabolism.

Two minutes of core-strengthening movements: This component of the workout includes two different exercises specifically targeted at the abdominal, back, and hip muscles.

One minute of stretching and breathing: The final minute oxygenates the cells, increases flexibility, and decreases stress.

The first four minutes of high-energy aerobic training are known as high-intensity interval training, which has been proven to be highly effective in burning calories. The initial two minutes function as a warm-up period, and through the full four-minute cycle you generate a significant caloric burn that greatly exceeds what you might get on a treadmill.

"When you're on a treadmill walking for 30 or 45 minutes, you look down at the little caloric expenditure and it says you burned a whopping 150 or maybe 200 calories. High-intensity interval training increases your heart rate to a level that you couldn't sustain for a long period of time. Then you lower your heart rate, coming back down to a moderate level."

In the process of this interval work, repeatedly increasing and decreasing your heart rate, you burn a lot of fat, but that's not all.

"As a result of your four-minute interval workout, we have found from scientific evidence that you increase your metabolic rate anywhere from 16–38 hours *after* the activity. This is what is called EPOC, or excess postexercise oxygen consumption. It's really the after-burn that is creating these incredible results."

Sean and his group have found that the four-minute, high-intensity interval sequence is effective for everyone from couch potatoes to elite athletes. Everyone has different start points in terms of their existing fitness levels, but interval training meets you where you are, allowing you to train as hard or as lightly as you want according to your existing level of conditioning. Doing this is simple and requires almost no gear: You can do it on a treadmill or stair-climber, or by alternating sprinting with jogging, or with a jump rope, or any other activity that gets your heart rate humming.

The next phase is three minutes of what Sean calls CREATE—compound resistance exercise and thermic effect.

"We've created resistance-training exercises that use multiple joints, where we're engaging multiple muscles in performing one to two exercises at a time. I'll give you an example. Almost everyone knows what a squat is. They are a great exercise for the front of the leg, the quadriceps, the hamstring, and the buttocks. However, we've designed an exercise that incorporates a squat, an arm curl, and a shoulder press. This accelerates the metabolic rate again, but it also hits multiple joints, and it hits multiple muscle groups as well.

"You need the biggest bang for your buck time-wise, and the way to do that is to maximize muscle and joint movements."

Everyone can do this by focusing attention on several simultaneous movements, working major muscle groups in tandem, for just three minutes per day!

The next step focuses on core strength, which is absolutely key to graceful aging. For two minutes you work exclusively on your abdominal, lower back, and hip muscles before finishing the program with one minute of dynamic stretching, incorporating deep breathing and stretching simultaneously. This minute also gives you recovery time if you wish to repeat the 4-3-2-1 circuit again.

At the peak of my fitness as a marathon runner and triathlete, I was accustomed to training far in excess of these numbers on a daily basis. As a 50-plus triathlete, still competing, looking to maintain my basic fitness levels and keep off excess weight, I have seen the incredible benefits of Sean's compressed exercise program. All of us must maintain a solid level of fitness, and this is the approach that will ensure you achieve that goal regardless of your busy schedule. As you become accustomed to regular exercise, you can also choose to repeat an entire 10-minute circuit, or portions of it, for an additional challenge and even better results.

"We have elite athletes in colleges right now who are doing the 4-3-2-1 program and we're seeing *amazing* results. Phenomenal changes in their aerobic endurance, cardiovascular endurance, their anaerobic endurance, their body composition, their strength—all of these areas are improving. What we're finding is that circuit training works: Moving from one exercise to another not only helps the cardiovascular system and your body's ability to burn calories—but also, for those of us who get bored easily (and we're all a little ADD when it comes to exercise), this is a perfect workout. It addresses all of the main barriers that we all struggle with—not only lack of time, but also our lack of confidence that we can successfully complete a regular workout. Anybody can do 10 minutes of exercise!"

Through ongoing testing and research, Sean has found that people using the 10-Minute Total Body Makeover achieve significant health benefits in a very short time. He has seen individuals make significant gains in cardiovascular health, weight loss, and body chemistry simply by doing a 10-minute workout three times a week for 12 weeks.

The program has been tested with children and adults of all ages, and it's flexible enough to accommodate virtually everyone. That means the whole family can get involved, even your kids. Sean's previous book was with Dr. William Sears—*LEAN Kids*—and one of the reasons he came up with the 4-3-2-1 program was to create something that would be effective for every age group.

"Kids don't want to do long, arduous aerobic activity. You won't see a child on a treadmill going for 30 or 45 minutes at a time, but what kids will do quite naturally are stop-and-start activities. It's interval training! I began to look at high-intensity interval training—really seeing the impact on not only metabolic rates, but also on weight management, fitness levels, body composition, blood chemistry, energy levels, and cardiovascular endurance. We began to test kids with this, and they loved it. They love to sprint and then stop, sprint and then stop, and we realized that adults really should be training like this as well. We've worked with individuals from eight years old all the way to 80 years old with this program."

In monitoring the progress of his clients, Sean has witnessed another dimension to working out that is just as important as the physical changes. He sees people experiencing significant benefits in their mental outlook, their emotional lives, their relationships, and even their spiritual life. This points yet again to the integrated nature of our wellness as human beings: The body affects the mind, emotions, and the spirit.

"Really, I think my favorite results are the mental, spiritual, and relational aspects of becoming fit. Our research has determined that motion affects *emotion*. If I can get somebody moving, they actually begin to change other areas of their life. They begin to eat differently, they begin to think differently, they begin to behave differently. We've even had people come back and tell us that their relationships are better, their spiritual lives are better. . . . Movement itself is a huge catalyst."

This type of research, describing the positive effects of exercise on mental and emotional health, is becoming increasingly well established in the medical literature. Studies are steadily emerging that show that even relatively low levels of weekly exercise create improvements in mood states, reduce anxiety, and improve self-esteem. I can certainly vouch for this. I know that when I occasionally neglect my own fitness training, my moods are more variable and my mental acuity suffers. The moral of the story is: We all need regular physical exercise to stay lean and feel good in body, mind, and soul. Almost all of us have found it difficult to always get to a gym or to find the time to do the physical activity our bodies require each week, but not anymore. No excuses with Sean's program. Now you know the importance of staying lean, and you also have the most cutting-edge plan for getting and staying physically fit (And you've got the plan first—so get a head start). Get moving!

INCREASING VITALITY AT EVERY AGE

chapter 9

with DR. MICHAEL ROIZEN

Dr. Michael Roizen is the director of wellness at the Cleveland Clinic and the cofounder of RealAge.com, a leading website that provides guidance on slowing aging through diet and lifestyle. He is the renowned author and coauthor of several

To slow your aging process and ensure optimal health, adopt a deeply committed attitude and observe this list of simple daily supplements and habits.

best-selling books on health and antiaging, including the *New York Times* number one best-selling *You: Staying Young* and *You: The Owner's Manual*, both coauthored with Dr. Mehmet Oz, with their new *You: Being Beautiful* appearing in autumn 2008.

Optimizing your body's health and increasing its vitality through nutrition and supplementation can boast few authorities as great as the inimitable Dr. Michael Roizen, America's expert on staying young. Mike's important message in all of his work is that most of us know less about the workings of our bodies than we should, and it's easy to add years to our lives and quality to our living through simple practices of daily exercise, diet, supplementation, regular sleep, and relaxation. Reducing your risk factors for major illnesses such as cancer and heart disease increases life expectancy by just under a decade, but Mike also provides insights into other components of bodily health so you can increase your life expectancy, rejuvenate your body, and get more out of living right *now*.

Mike is the living, breathing embodiment of what he preaches about antiaging medicine, so I couldn't help asking him what *his* real age is. In January 2008, Mike was 62 calendar years of age. However, according to biological measures, his "real age" at that time was about 42.5. Numerous practices and healthy habits have helped him to reduce his biological age by 20 years.

"There are 147 things men can do to keep themselves from aging. I do all of the simple things I talk about, like flossing regularly and taking triple-D— vitamin D3—and DHA in the right amounts.

"I don't eat saturated fat or trans fat, not even on my birthday. I try to avoid red meat all but once a month at most, and I've actually got it down to much less than that. If I'm going to eat grains, it's 100 percent whole grain—that is, 100 percent whole wheat, or rye, or whatever. I don't eat any processed foods. And, of course, I talk to you, which keeps laughter in my life!" says Mike.

Mike is in better health in his sixties than many of us are in our forties because he understands the little things that promote optimal health. He has written about 147 health habits for staying young, but there are four scientifically proven, extraordinarily simple daily supplements that he especially recommends to help you to live a longer, healthier life. He also identifies a couple of basic exercise and lifestyle habits that can prove very effective in adding quality years to your life. All of his recommendations are simple little things you can do every day to bolster your physical health, and they are easy to integrate into your general dietary and nutritional program.

The first thing Mike recommends for everyone is vitamin D3, what he likes to call "triple D," a substance that research shows to have incredible cancer-prevention powers. It's easy to take it daily and it's common at your local grocery store, pharmacy, or health food store. For optimal health and cancer prevention, Mike advises that we take 1,000 IU (international units) daily.

"We've really increased the amount of D3 that people should take. We used to recommend it for preventing rickets in bones, and it does that at 40–60 IU. About a year or two ago, the official powers in the United States—meaning the Institute of Medicine, the FDA, the USDA, and the HHS— increased the recommendation to 400 IU, but there has been a push to get it up to 1,000 IU per day because of the data on its prevention of cancer."

Is it possible to encounter toxicity at these levels? Researchers have determined that you can get up to 10,000 IU per day before toxicity becomes a concern, so you've got a pretty safe level at 1,000. The Canadian Pediatric Society even recommends 2,000 IU daily for pregnant and breast-feeding women. To get 1,000–2,000 IU, you most likely have to take your D3 in supplements because you won't find food with high enough concentrations other than cod-liver oil.

One of the most important tasks of vitamin D3 is to turn on what Mike calls a "spell-checker," which monitors our body's cell-duplication process. This is the cancer-fighting aspect of vitamin D3: The spell-checker makes sure that new cells are built the way they ought to be, and that mutated cancer cells don't slip past security.

"We all have a spell-checker that checks all our cell duplications. Our bodies have more than 300 million duplications a day. If you have enough vitamin D3 in your system to turn on your spell-checker, instead of turning a mis-duplication into a cancer, you kill it.

"It also decreases other immune-related and autoimmune diseases now thought to be related to thyroid deficiency in older people, as well as a number of other things, but the key strengths of vitamin D3 are cancer prevention and, of course, the prevention of rickets and bone disease."

The second thing that Mike recommends for everyone is docosahexaenoic acid, or DHA, an omega-3 essential fatty acid (so called because it cannot be produced within the body and must be acquired through diet). It decreases the risk of heart disease, decreases the risk of memory loss and Alzheimer's disease, and, according to recent research, probably decreases the risk of nervous system disease as well.

DHA is a healthy fat found in fish oil, so if you were to take cod-liver oil on a daily basis, you could get both your vitamin D3 and your DHA from that one source. The now-defunct tradition of mothers giving their children a healthy dose of cod-liver oil every day was actually grounded in this science, even if they weren't schooled in molecular biology and chemistry.

To get a sufficient daily dosage of DHA, you probably need to get it in pill form, in a capsule, or as a fish oil. If you don't like the smell or the risk of heavy-metal toxicity, which might be a concern with fish and fish oils, you can also get your DHA from where the fish get it—algae. (The International Fish Oil Standards progam (IFOS) rates fish oils for potency and purity. The website is www.ifosprogram.com.) There are a number of manufactured supplements that extract DHA from algae. You can get vitamins or pills with DHA online or at health stores, and Mike says you should aim for 600 mg a day.

The importance of DHA relates to one of the hottest topics in the last 15 years: the role of omega-3 unsaturated fatty acids in the prevention of a host of different ailments. Deficiency in omega-3 increases risk for many diseases we associate with aging, including Alzheimer's, cancer, heart disease, stroke, and inflammatory and autoimmune diseases. It's also been shown that people deficient in omega-3s are more likely to suffer from depression, fatigue, ADD, and type 2 diabetes. We also know that omega-3s improve brain function and increase fat loss. Part of the key to getting proper amounts of omega-3 is the *ratio* of omega-6 to omega-3 fatty acids in our diets, and it is generally accepted that our Western diets are not maintaining the right ratio of the two.

"If you look back at history, until about 300 years ago, our diets were providing a ratio of about one to one omega-6 to omega-3," Mike explains. "With the harvesting of the feed grains, mainly corn and maize, the ratio in our diet went to about four to one. And it is only since the 1950s that we have changed that four-to-one ratio, and now we are someplace between 16 to one and 24 to one, depending on populations."

Researchers still aren't certain what the exact ratio of omega-6 to omega-3 should be, but they know it should be a lot lower than 16 or 24 to one. One of the world's authorities on essential fatty acids, Dr. Artemis Simopoulos, recommends a four-to-one ratio at most. The biggest sources of omega-6 in Western diets are poultry, eggs, cereals, nuts, baked goods, most vegetable oils, and a host of other oils such as corn, safflower, sunflower, soybean, hemp, borage, and evening primrose. If you are able to limit these in your diet, in combination with taking an omega-3 supplement, you will go a long way to restoring a better balance of omega-3 and omega-6 in your system.

"We do know that increasing DHA to a point where you get back to a four-to-one ratio decreases the risk of Alzheimer's disease, decreases learning disabilities, improves infant brains, and decreases macular degeneration and retinal destruction. We *think* it may have other benefits."

Some people are also trying to use flaxseed oil as a dietary source of DHA, but the research on flaxseed oil as a supplementary source of DHA is not conclusive. In fact, it suggests that your body converts only a little less than 4 percent of the flaxseed oil to DHA, and it's the DHA that has the strongest correlation with brain, eye, and heart health.

Mike recommends two more supplements for anyone who wants to slow aging. They are respectively known for fighting Alzheimer's disease and slowing the progressive aging of your arteries associated with heart disease and stroke, and one is also known for decreasing your cancer risk. These two items are as simple and common as they are powerful, and you probably have them somewhere in your kitchen right now. You've probably never regarded them as anything more than condiments: Say hello to mustard and tomato sauce.

Tomato sauce and mustard both have especially good properties for reducing the risk of many ailments associated with aging. The turmeric in mustard decreases your risk of Alzheimer's disease, and tomato sauce decreases the risk of aging in your arteries as well as your cancer risk. Turmeric is the highest known source of beta-carotene, an antioxidant that helps protect the liver from free radical damage and helps the body to metabolize fats by decreasing the fat-storage rate in liver fat cells. It's also good to know that curcumin, the active ingredient in turmeric, suppresses pain without harmful side effects. Recent findings indicate that 1,200 mg of curcumin has the same effect as taking 300 mg of some anti-inflamatory drugs. Lycopene is the active ingredient in tomatoes and it is actually four times more bioavailable in tomato paste than in fresh tomatoes. Its antioxidant properties cut the risk of heart disease by 29 percent. Expressed as a daily average, Mike recommends 1 teaspoon of mustard with turmeric per day, and 1 1/2 tablespoons of tomato sauce per day, but you don't have to get mustard and tomato sauce *every day*. You simply need to get 10 tablespoons of tomato sauce over the course of a week, and 7 teaspoons of mustard.

One more thing: Mike doesn't advocate having your mustard on a hotdog! That's a little like getting your vitamin C in your double margarita. But mustard generally goes well with some lean meats, and it's also excellent in homemade salad dressings, and is now available in capsule form, so there are other ways to get it into your diet. Tomato sauce is probably even easier to get into your diet through pasta sauces and other tomato dishes.

These four items—vitamin D3, DHA, mustard, and tomato sauce—are Mike's favorite dietary supplements for improving your vitality and longevity. In addition to these, he also recommends a few simple lifestyle habits for improving your vitality and keeping you younger than your calendar age. One of the most effective is flossing.

Flossing your teeth is one of the most important things you can do to maintain your health and youth. You need teeth to eat, and flossing is the best way to keep your teeth healthy. If you want to dramatically reduce your risk of tooth decay and periodontal disease, flossing is the way to go; most dentists consider it even more important than brushing. Surprisingly, the benefits of flossing don't end in your mouth: Flossing also reduces your risk of heart disease because it rids your mouth of bacteria associated with causing heart ailments and inflammation, so the next time you see your dental hygienist, pay attention to how you are supposed to floss and start flossing regularly. It may prevent you from needing dentures one day, or even ending up in hospital with a heart condition.

And don't forget your attitude has a significant role to play in all of your health practices, as attitude will largely determine how well you follow regimens for diet, supplements, and exercise. Similar to what Dr. Bernie Siegel says about the importance of joy and hope in overcoming illness, Mike suggests that a positive attitude plays a huge part in aging well and staying healthy, if for no other reason than how it affects our decision making regarding lifestyle and diet. For example, if you are deeply committed to improving your nutrition or reducing your cholesterol, you are much more likely to stay on a cholesterol-reduced diet or daily supplementation plan to meet your vitamin and mineral requirements and stay within your cholesterol limits. It will also mean that you are much more likely to show up at the track for your run or to get to the gym as you promised.

Mike's advice makes it simple for you to get on track with staying young and vital. Remember, to slow your aging process and ensure optimal health, adopt the right attitude and observe Mike's list of simple supplements and habits, which are fast and easy to do on a daily and weekly basis. Remember to take your vitamin D3, DHA, tomato sauce, and mustard; remember to floss your teeth regularly; and remember to keep active with frequent exercise. If you stick faithfully to Mike's advice, your body will remain healthier and more vital despite the inevitable advance into "older" calendar age.

In the next chapter, we'll take this process even further by looking at natural sources and plant remedies for further optimization of your bodily health with the expert on plant medicines, Chris Kilham.

USING PLANT MEDICINE

chapter 10

with CHRIS KILHAM

Chris Kilham is an author, educator, the host of "Medicine Trail" (shot on location around the world), and the founder of Medicine Hunter Inc. When he is not teaching ethnobotany at the University of Massachusetts at Amherst, he transforms into what CNN refers to as the "Indiana Jones of plant medicine," traveling the world in search of the most time-honored and proven herbal and plant remedies.

There have been hundreds of very good studies supporting centuries of use of a wide variety of beneficial herbal remedies.

While many people take the latest synthetic pharmaceuticals, Chris seeks out medicinal plants from India, China, Siberia, Brazil, Venezuela, Peru, the South Pacific, Hawaii, Lebanon, Syria, Thailand, Austria, Malaysia, and other exotic locales.

Even when we diligently follow the health and fitness advice offered by experts such as Dr. Pamela Peeke, Sean Foy, and Dr. Michael Roizen, there may still be occasions in our lives when we contract ailments or find ourselves operating at less than 100 percent—that's just part of living. The question is how we deal with less-than-optimal health or illness when it arises. If we decide to use medicinal remedies or supplements, we are quickly faced with a choice of what type of medicine or product to take: natural or synthetic. If you talk to Chris Kilham, he would advise you to choose natural whenever possible.

As America's renowned "Medicine Hunter," Chris champions the use of plant sources for medicines and supplements, and he stands at the forefront of the growing movement toward their use in promoting optimal health. In the face of a global pharmaceutical industry that counts for hundreds of billions of dollars in annual earnings, his cause is simple: Plant medicines are just as effective as the medicines synthesized by the big pharmaceutical companies, and they're a lot safer. Based on his research as an ethnobotanist around the world, Chris can tell you the name of a plant-based medicine or natural supplement that matches almost any health need that arises, so you can enjoy healing benefits while avoiding the serious side effects of many pharmaceutical products. In this chapter, he has been kind enough to give us a rundown of his favorite plant remedies and supplements. He describes a few essential standbys that you may already know, and he reveals some excellent recently discovered medicinal plants that are sure to become big names shortly in the treatment of pressing health issues treated most often with medicines: arthritis, inflammation in general, indigestion, depression, anxiety, high cholesterol, enlarged prostate, high blood pressure, and even the common cold.

Chris makes it his business to keep up with the latest in peer-reviewed science and research on the safety and efficacy of natural supplements and plant remedies. There have been hundreds of very good studies supporting centuries of use of a wide variety of beneficial herbal remedies, and today there are tens of millions of Americans who benefit from taking natural supplements. With researchers like Chris traveling the globe looking for other plants, those numbers continue to grow. Chris points to the latest research into plant-based medicines being conducted at distinguished institutions across the United States and elsewhere that have proven their healing capabilities. The important news is that again and again, herbal medicines are proving to be safer alternatives to often dangerous pharmaceuticals.

"For example, you've heard a lot about the dangers of the anti-inflammatory drugs like Celebrex and Vioxx. Columbia University Medical Center and other very distinguished medical centers have done human studies on anti-inflammatory products that are entirely herbal, containing very concentrated extracts of ginger and turmeric. In those studies, they show significant anti-inflammatory activity without any—absolutely *none*—of the negative side effects associated with the pharmaceutical prescription anti-inflammatories."

If you are looking for safe anti-inflammatory medicine, there are exceptional plant-based sources that have already helped thousands of people. One source Chris recommends is turmeric, echoing Michael Roizen's fondness for the herb; the others are garlic and hops-extract products.

"There's a very good, clinically studied product on the market called Zyflamend that is available in natural food stores. It's undergone thorough clinical study at Columbia University Medical Center. There's also a hops-derived anti-inflammatory called FlexAgility MAX, which demonstrates outstanding anti-inflammatory activity without side effects. It's also available in natural food stores, so people *can* get relief from inflammation and do it in a natural way, and not face the potentially life-threatening side effects of drugs like Vioxx."

There's also solid research proving the effectiveness of plant medicines for the treatment of enlarged prostate, a condition that affects most men during their lifetime. Officially known as benign prostatic hyperplasia (BPH), enlarged prostate risk increases steadily after age 40. It affects 20 percent of men in their fifties, 60 percent of men in their sixties, and 70 percent of men by age 70. If a man develops an enlarged prostate, his chances are 25 percent that he will eventually require treatment—that's more than 350,000 men each year in the United States alone!

"We know that while Proscar is the most widely taken medical drug for enlarged prostate, extracts of saw palmetto, which is a palm fruit from the southeastern United States, have been shown to be every bit as effective and completely side effect-free in human clinical studies."

In the U.S., anxiety disorders affect 40 million adults age 18 and older, accounting for more than $42 billion a year in treatment costs. When it comes to treating anxiety disorders, there are also alternatives to the common pharmaceutical solutions.

"We know that the benzodiazepine drugs like Xanax, Serax, and Valium have grave side effects," Chris points out. "Many people have died from them, they're addictive, and in some cases they cause hallucinations and very serious psychological disorders. According to the Duke University Medical Center, kava extract is every bit as effective as those drugs for the treatment of anxiety, but is safer and has none of the negative effects. They have also found it completely safe for the liver."

Chris advocates another plant remedy that is commonly used to combat mental and emotional unease: St. John's wort. If you suffer from mild to moderate depression, St. John's wort is a herbal remedy that has been widely tested and well proven after centuries of use in Europe, dating back to ancient Greece.

"There are at this point in time hundreds of examples of products like the *very* well-proven St. John's wort or dozens of other herbs, such as echinacea, which reduces the duration and severity of a cold. All of these things have been proven by clearing the highest bar you can set in science."

I spoke with Chris the day after a particular self-styled medical writer appeared on national television in the United States, alleging that there was no science backing the efficacy of herbal remedies. Chris was characteristically vociferous in his response.

"Of course, the science on herbs is wide and vast and deep, which is why the World Health Organization has books about herbal medicines. Our medical writer friend says there are no manufacturing guidelines because he's completely unaware of the close to 20 or so federal and state statutes by which *all* supplement manufacturers have to operate.

"He says that people don't get results, even though the clinical efficacy of botanical medicines is very well established in double-blind, placebo-controlled, human clinical studies— the exact same kinds of studies that are used to demonstrate efficacy for prescription and over-the-counter drugs."

If you have any doubts about the efficacy of plant medicines and supplements, you might enjoy taking a little time to read some of the studies conducted by institutions such as Columbia University Medical Center and Duke University Medical Center, many of which are accessible through reputable health magazines and even online journals. The concern for anyone who cares about natural health is that misinformation about plant-source medicines and supplements may otherwise be taking away hope for millions of people who have tried dangerous, expensive, and potentially life-threatening drugs and now want to turn to safer natural alternatives instead.

All the while, it's inspiring to know that there are always more natural options coming to light. Many recently discovered plants and herbs are just now being brought to the commercial market. Based on his most recent explorations around the world, Chris offers a number of exciting predictions concerning which plants will be the most popular in the coming years.

"In terms of hot plants, we're going to see more appreciation for some of the old favorites," says Chris. "I think that as *Rhodiola rosea* gets even better established for its psychiatric uses, like treating certain cases of depression and other disorders, we're going to see it continue to grow in popularity."

Dr. Pamela Peeke highlighted the fact that we need to keep our bodies' stress response low in order to avoid the accumulation of toxic fat. Chris identifies a particular family of plants that can help if you're subjected to a lot of mental and emotional stress: He suggests you investigate the adaptogen herbs as they are very effective in controlling blood cortisol levels.

"I think that the market for adaptogens, the class of herbs that strengthen you overall and help to ward off stress, will continue to grow. There's a plant that I am particularly fond of called holy basil, which significantly lowers cortisol, the primary stress hormone in the blood, and it makes people feel very good. Even though it has been available in the North American market for a couple of years now, I think we're going to see a big jump in holy basil's popularity this year as it becomes further established and people discover how it improves their mood immediately."

Chris is also excited about the potential of maca, a root from the Andes of Peru, which he thinks will become much more widely used this year as it appears in many mass-market venues for the first time. Maca root (*Lepidium meyenii*) is a native plant resembling a turnip or radish that grows in poor soil at high altitude under some of the most extreme cold conditions on earth. It has been cultivated above 14,000 feet by Andean peoples as a primary food staple for over 2,000 years, and it is known to enhance energy, endurance, stamina, and sexual function. It's also a sustainable crop that helps local Peruvians escape poverty and the dangers of mining work.

"The popularization of maca has enabled many people in the central highlands of Peru to earn a living cultivating this traditional crop. It has also provided an alternative to working in the mines, which are horrible places where people die young. The maca boom in the central highlands has given hope to many."

One of Chris's favorite recent discoveries is acai (pronounced *ah-sigh-ee*), a dark purple berry from the Amazon basin with strong antioxidant properties.

"Acai is a purple palm fruit. Purple fruits like blueberry and elderberry and some of the other berries have gotten a lot of attention over the past few years because what makes them purple are these tremendously powerful antioxidant compounds called anthocyanins.

"The more purple the better, and acai is the most purple of them all. It has the highest value of these pigments, and therefore has the highest antioxidant activity of any known fruit. Not only is it delicious, it also has absolutely superior body-protective properties. It actually protects your cells from destruction, and I think this exemplifies the Hippocratic expression 'Use your food as your medicine.' There are so many powerful medicinal foods—garlic, ginger, hot chilies, tea—and this is one of the really big ones."

With the plethora of proven and tested natural remedies available to us, you might find it astonishing how much negative reporting continues to appear in the popular press about herbal plant-based medicine. But there are billions of dollars to be made with prescription medications, so there's bound to be a turf war. Advertising budgets at the big pharmaceutical companies are geared accordingly, commanding plenty of television prime time and full-page ads in major magazines. Along the way, the occasional self-proclaimed medical pundit slamming the herbal industry helps to sway public opinion as well. That's all part of the public relations game.

As the battle rages, it's remarkable to consider that some of the most famous medications in history have been plant-based, including those produced by the big pharmaceutical companies. When Aspirin was introduced by Bayer in the early 1900s, they were using the substance found in the bark of the white willow tree as their main ingredient.

"Salicin from white willow led to the development of what we know as Aspirin." Chris points out. "Many of the medicines that are still in use today are plant-derived, and some of them have created a really big splash recently, like Taxol, for example, which is extracted from a tree and used to treat breast cancer. There are so many things—blood pressure medications, blood-thinning agents, cardiovascular enhancers like digitalis and digitoxin—that come from common garden plants. There are many drugs derived solely from plants that are actually among our safest and most effective medications."

Problems with medicinal toxicity seem to begin when we start *tinkering* with chemistry by developing new molecules that have never existed in nature before. Part of the argument for herbal and plant medicines is that these types of toxicity issues are greatly reduced because we're often using remedies that have been used and proven safe for centuries, versus synthetic pharmaceuticals that have had relatively few years of use and clinical trials.

"I think that the pharmaceutical industry is very annoyed with natural remedies," says Chris. "And from time to time, I do think they are involved in some of the negative stories that defame the reputation of plant-based medicines. They definitely have a significant agenda. They don't want something like kava to be used in place of Valium, because Valium is worth a billion dollars. Look at what just happened with Zyprexa. For 10 years the folks at Pfizer hid the fact that it caused obesity and diabetes. They allowed bipolar people to be on this dangerous drug, and increased their risk of a host of other health disorders."

As Chris says, there's a significant level of dishonesty and skullduggery in Big Pharma as there is whenever billions of dollars change hands. Intrigue and deceit are not unique to the pharmaceutical sector, but it certainly forms a very powerful part of the market. Taken as a whole, it makes Big Pharma a tough entity to fight, and it means that proponents of natural medicine may have a battle on their hands for the foreseeable future.

While the struggle continues, you can still avail yourself of some of the many fine plant-based remedies and natural super-foods that are available on the market today. When I last talked with Chris, I asked him to offer a top 10 list of his favorite medicinal plants and vital foods—a kind of "If you were trapped on a desert island and you could have nothing else" list. You can use most of these on a daily basis to greatly enhance your health and vitality without worrying that you are taking too much.

"I would unquestionably take the adaptogenic herbs," says Chris. "Adaptogens enhance endurance, stamina, strength, alertness, mental function, and immunity, and they help you to utilize oxygen better. My top four adaptogen herbs are schizandra berry, *Rhodiola rosea*—my favorite of all botanicals—eleuthero root, which used to be called Siberian ginseng, and the Indian herb ashwaghanda. While ashwaghanda has an almost imponderable name from a spelling standpoint, it is a great adaptogenic herb. When you take it, you feel good.

"For inflammation, colds, and general digestive purposes, I would absolutely bring ginger root with me because I find it to be one of the most versatile healers. Whether you've eaten a little too much, you're coming down with a cold, or you've got sinus congestion, you just have to shred up some ginger root and make a tea out of it to feel better. That's quite remarkable.

"Since I'm over 50 and should probably be paying attention to what's happening with my cholesterol, I would definitely bring garlic with me. The body of science about garlic goes on forever. I like the flavor, and in terms of lowering bad LDL cholesterol, improving HDL cholesterol, and reducing high blood pressure, it's one of the best natural remedies we have.

"I'd also bring along green tea. As common and widely discussed as it is, green tea is still one of the best, most effective, and least expensive of all the natural remedies we have. I drink a couple of cups every night. For its cholesterol-lowering benefits, its anticancer properties, and its protective qualities against UVA and UVB rays, I would have to put it on the list.

"And I would definitely want to bring along acai. I don't exactly call this a herb, but I think it's a super-food that gets treated like a herb.

"Finally, I'd bring along some really impressive immune enhancers to round out nature's pharmacy. I'd bring reishi mushroom, which has a long history of traditional use, and a *growing* history of conventional use and scientific analysis for reducing the risk of cancer and helping the recovery of chemotherapy sufferers. I would also include cat's claw, the Amazonian herb, in my medicinal trick bag because it balances the immune system. It brings low immune function up to a higher level, and it brings overly high immune function down to a normal healthy level. It also has cancer-fighting properties, and it's very good for things like allergies. It's a powerful anti-inflammatory."

You can take schizandra, *Rhodeola*, eleuthero, ashwaghanda, ginger root, garlic, green tea, and acai every single day. It's just good sense to add them to your personal biology to keep you healthy and disease free. When you have a cold or flu, or are dealing with compromised immune function, add reishi mushroom and cat's claw. Chris recommends using cat's claw sparingly and only for medicinal treatment purposes.

"You can use reishi often, but not cat's claw. Cat's claw should be treated like ibuprofen. I mean, you don't get up every day and say, 'Well, I'll just belt back a couple of Advils and then hopefully I won't experience any pain.' You would be more likely to use something like that if you *felt* pain, so cat's claw is one of the two conspicuous exceptions to daily consumption."

Stock your plant-based medicine cabinet with Chris's top 10 list: schizandra berry, *Rhodeola rosea* root, eleuthero, the Indian herb ashwaghanda, fresh ginger root, fresh garlic, green tea, acai berry, reishi mushrooms, and cat's claw. If you are ever prescribed pharmaceuticals for a condition, proceed with extreme caution, especially if it's a recently developed drug, and don't be afraid to ask your doctor about possible side effects. Consider using a plant-based medicine under direction from a qualified naturopath, herbalist, or pharmacist who is knowledgeable about natural medicine, and use some of Chris's recommended plants for daily health maintenance and enhanced vitality. This is your body, and you choose what you put into it.

We've done much to address the health needs of your body through the advice of Dr. Pamela Peeke, Sean Foy, Dr. Michael Roizen, and Chris Kilham. In our next five chapters, we'll move beyond the physical body toward a discussion of its higher purpose for being: living a rich mental and spiritual life that is both given expression and mediated through this physical vessel of flesh and bone.

SECTION 3

What is spirit, and how do we come to know our own? In the following chapters, I'll introduce you to some of today's leading spiritual teachers and authors who have appeared on *The Good Life* to tell the story of their own spiritual transformations. Along the way, you will discover their suggestions for nurturing a rich and inspiring life for your soul that will infuse your body and mind with new vigor and purpose.

Implicit in spiritual living is the understanding that there is a source or power greater than the narrow physical bounds of "self" that our mind perceives, and this source exists whether or not our mind comprehends it or even acknowledges its existence. The

HEALTH OF SPIRIT

spirit cannot be completely defined with mere words: It must be experienced. The mind plays an intermediary role in leading our daily spiritual practices and habits, but its perceptual power stops at the threshold of the spiritual realm.

In these final five chapters, you will discover important ways of examining the life of your soul. While none of the following authors and teachers are orthodox religionists, all of them reflect upon time-tested spiritual practices and habits that are familiar to the sagely traditions of many faiths. You will find the experience and wisdom they offer uplifting and inspiring in your own spiritual life, and will complete your circle of health in body, mind, and spirit.

FINDING YOUR
CALLING
chapter 11

with AZIM JAMAL

Azim Jamal is a leading inspirational speaker, management consultant, and executive coach. He made his life-changing career switch from "accounting for business" to "accounting for life" during a soul-stirring experience while volunteering in the developing world. Overcome by the plight of homeless refugees in war-torn areas, he vowed to make a difference in

Many of us leave this earth with our song still in us.

people's lives. Since then, Azim has been spreading his unique, thought-provoking message in becoming a Corporate Sufi—one who can achieve material abundance through spiritual abundance. Azim is the author of several books, including the number one Amazon best-selling *The Power of Giving*. Over 1 million people worldwide have heard his inspiring words, and his work has received accolades from leading thinkers, including Dr. Deepak Chopra, Dr. Wayne Dyer, Jack Canfield, Brian Tracy, and Dr. Ken Blanchard.

Do you pay much attention to the health of your soul? For many people, their daily activities are guided by their spiritual sensitivities and beliefs, and the routines of their lives include spiritual practices that enhance and energize their activities. For others, the soul is merely an abstract idea that they are seldom aware of, and whose role in their lives is essentially discounted. Some never have an inkling of the life of their spirit until they have an experience that shocks them into a sudden discovery of a deeper world within themselves, one beyond the bounds of their daily physical habits and mental calibrations.

Somewhere between these two scenarios is where Azim Jamal found himself when he took a volunteer posting as an accountant in the developing world some years ago. Azim is now known as a leading inspirational speaker, management consultant, and executive coach who has earned the title of the "Corporate Sufi," but he came to his current vocation by virtue of a shock to his spiritual system during a fateful volunteer trip overseas. In the story of how he went from being a straitlaced corporate accountant to being St. Francis with a spreadsheet, you will find fresh insight into how to invigorate your own spiritual life with a new sense of purpose in this world.

"I changed from accounting for business to accounting for life when I had a soul-stirring experience while doing voluntary work in the developing world in 1997. I was so moved by what I saw that my life was never the same again."

If you can imagine yourself in his place, you'll see how his experience could shock a person into a completely new life orientation and outlook. In the dusty backstreets of Pakistan's capital, Karachi, Azim was confronted by scenes of such sublime human dignity amid unfathomable suffering that it completely reoriented his sense of direction and purpose.

"I interviewed about 14 Afghan refugees in a small hut. I asked them questions about how much money they needed to live on, and I heard stories of the family going from war to war to war; of the children having never gone to school; of how they fled from Kabul, Afghanistan, to go to Karachi, walking for 19 days in the mountains in cold weather with just the shirts on their backs. Some of them didn't have any shoes to wear, some of them got sick in the mountains, but still they had to walk, otherwise they would die. Some women gave birth to children in those mountains. Eventually they made it to Karachi.

"Several of them worked in the hot blazing sun for 14 hours a day, selling corn on a trolley, making a dollar a day, which didn't even pay the rent for the small hut. I saw young kids holding a piece of bread as if their life was at stake. In the midst of this, somehow they were able to offer me dried fruit, because I was a guest."

The staggering contrast between their squalor and their generosity proved overwhelming for Azim. Sitting with them in that hut, his emotions quickly overcame him to the degree that he began to have a physical reaction. He started to feel sick. He felt so sick, in fact, that he simply had to get up and leave in the middle of the interview.

"As I walked out of the hut, the whole village looked at me because I was wearing a suit," says Azim. He recounts this part of the experience with a tone that blends self-loathing with frustration at the pathos of the scene. "And I saw mostly women and children because the men had died. I saw children with rosy cheeks and big eyes, and a smile on their faces despite their plight. I was there no more than 20 or 30 seconds, but it seemed like eternity to me, and I couldn't take it anymore. I was totally shattered.

"So I went to the cab that was waiting for me, and I went back to my hotel. In the back of the cab I was crying, shivering, and sweating at the same time, despite the hot weather."

In the 25 minutes that it took to return to the hotel, Azim says something happened to his soul.

"I call it my defining moment. Since then, my life has never been the same."

That was the moment that Azim decided to make the shift from being a professional accountant with three degrees to sharing a message of giving and the power behind it. His experience with the refugees eventually led him to write *The Power of Giving* and to speak widely on the theme of living a charitable life. His book describes the lessons of his defining moment, as well as something even more fundamental that he has learned since that day in Karachi: the importance of finding a life balance among money, family, health, and spirit.

Life balance forms the essence of being what Azim calls a "Corporate Sufi," wherein your life encompasses the themes of physical, mental, and spiritual well-being within a healthy, holistic life. ("Sufi" is a reference to the ancient tradition of Muslim mystics who wore simple robes of wool, or *soof*, as a symbol of simplicity, humility, and purity.) Azim is interested in how we can align our daily activities in the world of family and work with our highest spiritual aspirations or calling in life. In his book *Life Balance the Sufi Way*, coauthored with Nido Qubein, Azim talks about managing a balance between your spiritual needs and your material life shaped by your career and family. If you find yourself overwhelmed by living in the hectic workaday world that Yossi Ghinsberg described earlier, and if you hold any notion that there could be a spiritual life beyond company lunch meetings, working weekends, car payments, and the occasional vacation, Azim's message will be timely for you.

"One of the biggest struggles people are having in corporations is that they get burned out. They can't sustain their success. They're finding it's much too one-sided, meaning there's change in material success, but you're finding something empty at the end. There's no balance between materiality and spirituality."

"Corporations are all about success, about ambition, about power and material abundance. Sufism is about looking at the essence, not the form, and being grounded in principles, values, ethics—living in the power of giving, living in the moment, and living in spiritual abundance."

In short, the approach of the Corporate Sufi is to manage a marriage of these contrasting worlds of matter and spirit. We have to live in this world and pay the mortgage even while feeding our spirits and helping those around us, so we need to practise lifestyle habits and contemplative techniques that help us to nurture that balanced union. And what happens when a person successfully balances material ambition with spiritual aspiration? You get someone who is efficient, motivated, and goal-oriented in the pursuit of material abundance, but this pursuit remains heart-centered and balanced with the observation of spiritual principles and ethics.

"It's not just about having equal time for body, mind, spirit. It's more than that. It's time management, self-management, and energy management—being able to manage your energy, and doing what you love to do. In this way, you're going to be less tired, and you're able to get more for the amount of effort that you're putting in. When you know your priorities well and stay centered in that knowledge, then you're able to make decisions that consistently maintain your highest principles, your highest priorities."

So how do you achieve that? How do you *find* what you love to do, and how do you *do* what you love to do? It might seem easier said than done, and Azim acknowledges that it is difficult, or at least that it's rare. He offers some advice on how to find your calling, your principles, your priorities, and then integrate them into your life and work.

"It's really a question of awareness, a question of observation. People *see* things, but they don't *observe*.

"If you observe yourself every day, and if you're very particular about it, you'll find some moments of magic. You'll discover and notice those moments when you feel really energetic.

"Stop and ask: What am I doing now? Why do I feel this kind of peace inside me? And if you keep observing, you'll get a glimpse of what you're all about—what really makes you tick, what really excites you, what makes you really passionate."

I can identify with what Azim says as I have learned to observe and recognize this sensation in my own life.

Sometimes, in the middle of an interview, I will suddenly have a profound, deep sensation as I listen to my guest speak. My brain and my heart seem to tingle as I sense the inspirational power of the message. It was when I first tuned into this sensation that I realized the direction, the *right* direction, of my life. Strange as it may sound, in that suspended moment, I can sense the impact of the interview on the listeners. It's in that moment that I most strongly feel the passion in what I do, and I even garner a sense that I might be fulfilling a small part of some larger good work in this world.

"Another way of tuning into yourself is to ask yourself what you would do—what kind of work would you do—if you won a lottery today. Then you ask yourself: Am I doing it for the money? Or am I doing it because I really need to? If you clear away the issues that can surround money, what would you do? That will open the way for you to see what is really important for you."

Would I still conduct interviews if I had $40 million in my savings account? Absolutely, and I'd probably have time to do more interviews and write more books. What would you do? Try to picture yourself with bags of money, where financial concerns would no longer be an obstacle to what you choose to do in your daily life, and then imagine what you would choose to do. What would it be? Be prepared. The images that come to you might be surprising. You might discover that your dream is to be a commercial fisherman, an airline pilot, a preschool teacher, a broadcaster, a scuba instructor, an artist, or any one of 1,000 things you've never permitted yourself to consider.

"If today was your last day, and you looked back at your life, what's the one regret you'll have?" asks Azim. "When you reflect on that, you'll get a perspective very different from what you have now. It will tell you what you were born to do, but haven't done yet. This is the key."

This reminds me of speaking with Dr. Wayne Dyer on *The Good Life*. He said that many of us leave this earth with our song still in us. Does that ring any bells for you? If it does, even a little bit, then there's something vital for you to examine—a small voice that needs to grow loud and that needs to be heard. It doesn't necessarily mean that your life is completely off the rails; it means your soul is whispering to you that something is missing in your life. You can change that.

"The other way to really help you find your calling is, I believe, through meditation. We all grow tremendously from time spent in a quiet space, getting into our spirits, and in that quiet, you'll find moments of connection to your deepest self. You'll find out what you're here for."

Azim has been meditating since 1972, and he says his meditation practice has been a huge factor in shaping his life and work. He likes to meditate for about an hour every morning, and he wakes up very early to do it. While he misses some days, he figures he meditates about 90 percent of the mornings, and his meditation has been the one single factor that's helped him gain better insight into his life's purpose and also maintain his inner peace and happiness.

"In meditation, the fewer rules the better. Basically, you find a quiet space, where there is not much noise. The closer to nature the better—find a river, or trees, or somewhere near the ocean. Nature is inherently quiet, so it will lead you to become quiet."

It's also good to meditate in the early morning, when most people are still asleep, it's less noisy, and you have much less chance of being interrupted.

"And then become like a feather in the river—float. The feather never fights the river; it floats, so become like the feather. Thoughts will come, thoughts will go. Don't cling to any one thought because when you cling to one thought, you get into thinking mode. You want to just keep floating—let the thoughts come and go.

"That's it; that's meditation. If you do it for 10 minutes, or 20 minutes, or an hour, or whatever you feel comfortable with, if you get one second or even a millionth of a second of connection, that's enough. That's enough for you to really get a breakthrough, to feel that peace, that connection that is so powerful it is beyond words to describe."

As you develop your meditation practice and take time to reflect on your life on a regular basis, you will refine your capacity to make the kinds of discernments and decisions that are necessary to become a Corporate Sufi. Being a Corporate Sufi means being able to make decisions on a daily basis, and being able to execute them in an efficient, businesslike manner. This holds equally well for your personal and spiritual life as it does for your work life. Part of your decision making will come from goal setting, though Azim carefully qualifies what he means by "goals."

"I have goals. I have a vision, and I'm very specific," says Azim. "I'm number-oriented because I have a professional accounting background. However, the Sufi part of me makes me live in the moment, live for today. It reminds me to give everything that I have for today. If I can't align my action with my goals and my vision, then my vision and goals become nothing more than a hindrance. They take energy away from putting my efforts into today."

Azim is quick to add that "living in the moment" is a practice that many people speak about, but few master. "Most of us are too consumed by the past and future. We worry about what has already happened—things we cannot do much about. We worry about what needs to be done in the future or what could happen in the future, but no one knows what will happen in the future. At the end of the day, what will count is the execution in the moment."

The idea is not to force things. Maintaining your vision, work, and effort is different from trying to smash your way through to an objective. You have to maintain faith on those difficult days when it feels impossible to interweave your daily actions with your larger goals, and from there wait for the next opening or opportunity to align your life with your vision. As you do so, make sure you have defined both short-term and long-term goals.

"I have long-term goals, but I have to execute and implement them in the short term today, in the now. Then it becomes a good marriage of the two. When you're about to make a choice, ask yourself: Is it aligned to your bigger purpose? Is it aligned to your goals? Is it aligned to your vision? And sometimes this creates very difficult decisions. Stop and ask yourself: How is this decision going to help me with my mission? How is this decision going to help me with my vision? How is this decision going to help me with my goals? Then you're connecting to yourself all the time, and to me, that's incredibly powerful. It goes back to my model of the Corporate Sufi. The 'corporate' is the goal setting, the vision setting, the direction, and the 'Sufi' is the living in the moment, and executing in the moment, and connecting those two."

Azim's book, *The Power of Giving*, grew out of the renewed alignment of his values and his actions. In this case, the book talks about walking the walk when it comes to the virtue and value of giving, but it's also more. As Azim outlines in his book, there is a transformative *power* that takes hold when we give. As we have heard time and time again, giving changes the giver.

Azim will tell you that people who haven't tasted the beauty of giving don't know what they're missing. He tells the story about a fund-raiser who goes to a rich man for a donation, and the rich man is adamant that he never gives money to anyone. The fund-raiser persists, but eventually he sees that the rich man is not budging, so the fund-raiser says, "Okay, give me the sand from the ground and I will go." The rich man is perplexed. He tells the fund-raiser the sand is free, and that he can take it himself, but the fund-raiser insists: He wants the rich man to give it to him, and then he'll leave. Because the rich man is getting tired of him persisting, he gives him the sand. The fund-raiser turns and starts to leave. The rich man is still confused, so he calls after the fund-raiser and asks him, "Why did you ask me for the sand?" And the fund-raiser responds, "I wanted you to taste the beauty of giving." He explains that even though it's only sand, the rich man has now gained a small taste for charity, and eventually he'll have the appetite to give something more.

From his travels worldwide speaking to thousands of people, Azim has seen many instances of unparalleled generosity in the least expected circumstances. In addition to his transformative experience with the Afghan refugees in Karachi, one compelling experience happened after he lost his travel bags in Turkey just prior to a two-day speaking engagement in Tajikistan, one of the world's poorest countries. He arrived in Tajikistan with only jeans and a T-shirt, and the next flight wasn't coming for three more days. There was no chance that he'd be getting his baggage and his dress clothes in time for his presentations, but he had to proceed with the first day of his seminar regardless.

"I did the seminar, and there was this guy who was wearing a nice sleek blue shirt," says Azim. "I commented to him, during break time, 'You're wearing a nice shirt.' The next day, this same fellow brought me a new shirt, the same kind of shirt that he was wearing—my size—and gave it to me as a gift. Now, we're talking about the poorest country in the world. That to me is richness."

As when the Afghan refugees offered him dried fruit years previously, Azim was awestruck that people living in poverty would spontaneously offer a gift of so much relative wealth. "They don't have much to give in material terms, but they really understand the practice of giving."

There are essential, immutable life principles behind the power of giving, and this is why giving is so important. We were made to be generous with one another, and when the flow of giving stops, we interfere with a fundamental mechanism of nature and the universe. As Azim points out, a cow that isn't milked will stop producing milk, a sheep that isn't sheared will stop producing wool, and a fruit tree that isn't picked will stop producing fruit. When we stop giving, we stop the flow of abundance that is meant to be shared within our communities, and we stagnate in both material wealth and spiritual wealth. Put another way, we stop *living* to our full capacity as human beings.

"When you're in the flow of giving, more giving flows to you. When you're in the flow of abundance, more abundance flows through you. And we have amazing things to give—all of us. Not necessarily money. It can be skills, it can be time, it can be energy, it can be a prayer. It could be many things. And the more we give, the more we find."

What do you have to give? You might find it's a fun exercise to sit down and make an inventory of your own wealth, monetary or otherwise. Imagine what happiness you might be able to bring someone through even a small share of your wealth or talents. I have a friend whose son is a talented pianist, and he plays free classical concerts in an old-age home. It costs him nothing more than an hour of his time, yet it brings joy to a large number of house-bound seniors who would otherwise be unable to enjoy the beauty of live performances of Mozart, Beethoven, and Chopin. Others donate their time as volunteers in free inner-city dental clinics or community programs serving children and youth. It doesn't have to be money that you give.

The first step is to reflect on what you value in life. Then align yourself with those ideas. Last, you take decisive action based on those values, in the manner of a Corporate Sufi.

"Start now. Whatever you want to do, begin now. Spend a few minutes to write a letter to yourself. Say to yourself: If I could do anything in my life, what would I want to do?"

And once you have a vision of your purpose, you will have all the power you need to do whatever it is you value, as long as you know what you truly want and focus on it. Don't listen to the critics around you. Know what you want, hold it in focus, and you will be able to implement your vision by executing the decisive action it requires on a daily basis. And as your vision and life work bear fruit, share the fruits and rewards with those around you. Turn it outwards in a sincere expression of giving, just as the Corporate Sufi would do.

REALIZING YOUR LIFE'S PURPOSE

chapter 12

with BOB PROCTOR

Bob Proctor is an author, lecturer, entrepreneur, and consultant at the forefront of the human potential movement promoting the power of positive thinking and the Law of Attraction. For 40 years, Bob Proctor has focused on helping people create lives of prosperity,

> *"There are two important days in your life. One is the day you're born, and the second is the day you decide why you were born."*

rewarding relationships, and spiritual awareness. Recently made famous for his appearance in the film *The Secret*, his teaching and practice is closely aligned with the writings and work of other luminaries in the field of positive thought and abundance, such as Napoleon Hill and Earl Nightingale. Bob Proctor now travels the globe, teaching thousands of people how to believe in and act upon the greatness of their own minds.

As Azim Jamal describes, to live a complete and balanced life, you need to hear the messages that your soul speaks, and from those messages make the choices that will allow you to realize your life purpose on earth. Life's ultimate achievement is to bring your guidance, life purpose, and actions into harmony so that you can shape the kind of rewarding life that you dream of—one that balances, body, mind, and soul.

A balanced, abundant, and rewarding life means different things to different people, but certainly one definition is to be able to make your living by finding and following your life's passion. There are large, universal laws that have a hand in shaping our lives around our passions, and one of the greatest masters of these laws is Bob Proctor.

Hundreds of millions of people worldwide have learned about the Law of Attraction through the phenomenally successful movie and book, *The Secret*. It features some of the world's leading authorities on the subject of positive thinking and the Law of Attraction, and perhaps foremost among them is Bob Proctor, the star of *The Secret*. For over four decades, Bob has been teaching the Law of Attraction and the steps we can take to make it work in our lives. Personally, I've been fortunate to enjoy his friendship and mentoring for the past 10 years, and to learn the principles from him firsthand.

There is an old saying that anyone who has studied martial arts knows well: When the student is ready, the teacher appears. I was well versed in broadcasting, but a neophyte in my understanding of universal laws when Bob Proctor appeared in my life in early 1997, taking on the role of my teacher, friend, and mentor. In many respects, if Bob hadn't come into my life when he did, I may never have had the courage or insight to do what I really wanted to do, so I owe much to Bob for teaching me the Law of Attraction.

According to Bob and other teachers of the Law of Attraction, we essentially attract money, careers, and desired relationships into our lives by planting firm, positive beliefs about these things within our subconscious. Conversely, we deny ourselves those experiences if our subconscious beliefs and thoughts don't acknowledge that such a reality is possible for us, so the first step in engaging the Law of Attraction is to *believe* that we can have those things.

The next steps are where the work happens. These may not appear earth-shattering, but they are as critical in importance as they are deceptive in their simplicity: discovering your life purpose, committing to a vision, and then making and following short- and medium-term goals to realize that vision.

I'd like to share some of my story with you because I think some of the ups and downs I experienced reflect the stories of many readers who have pursued their life goals and been met with adversity.

My story begins 30 years ago when I decided I wanted to work in broadcasting. I applied to work at a small radio station, and in short order I received a reply letter. The contents of the letter offered me little encouragement. The letter said in no uncertain terms that they wouldn't even think of hiring me in any capacity, not even for the all-night show.

If you've ever faced a major rejection in your life, you can imagine how deflated I felt.

But despite my rejection, I continued to pursue my radio broadcasting dream. I kept plugging away with applications, and eventually I was hired at a small radio station, and ecstatic to be on-air.

According to Bob, what happened next was a perfect example of the Law of Attraction at work: Within a couple of years, I was named on-air personality of the year nationwide in Canada, featured in a documentary as one of the top five radio personalities in the world, and won several broadcasting awards. As my career evolved over the last 15 years, it was Bob who helped me transform my career further by teaching me the intricacies of its principles.

Let's look at this in a different way. Have you ever been thinking about someone and the phone rings and it's that person? *Hey, I was just thinking about you.* Or, have you ever bumped into someone whom you haven't seen in years, and then oddly, you bump into the same person several more times over the next few days or weeks? You might begin to think, "Hmm . . . perhaps it's not a coincidence." As Dr. Joan Borysenko will discuss in our next chapter, perhaps you're being sent a message, and it's up to you to tune into the frequency and continue listening for the signals.

Many years ago, I had just such an experience of coincidence with Bob that would prove extremely influential in my life. At the time, I was working for myself, and focused on what I love: learning and teaching about health. I had received an offer to return to the radio broadcasting business and host a morning program at a station I worked at some years prior. The station was doing really well and said they'd love it if I'd consider coming back to host the morning show.

I politely said no. I explained that I was working on building a health and lifestyle-related business, and I wanted to continue pursuing it.

But they persisted, and they offered me more each time they contacted me—more money, more perks. It was beginning to tempt me. The truth was I was slowly becoming an entrepreneur and building my new health business, but the operative word was *slowly*. With the radio station offer, all I had to do was sign a contract and I would be back to earning the kind of living that I had enjoyed before I set out on my own ventures. I had gone from a comfortable lifestyle to earning relatively little, so a part of this offer was certainly attractive.

My wife, on the other hand, liked the new entrepreneurial me. She saw that I was more in tune with myself since leaving the world of big broadcasting, and as my best friend, I was inclined to trust her insight in this situation. Somewhere in the process of me saying no and the station becoming more persistent, I realized that this wasn't just about another radio gig: This was my career and my life on the line.

As you can imagine, I had to contend with some serious mental pressures in my decision. I had a deep and honest realization that if I said no to this offer, there wouldn't be any more. This was it. I was going to say goodbye to my 25-year career and venture forth on my own, or I was going to get back on the merry-go-round of being an employee again, dancing to the beat of someone else's drum. It wasn't easy.

Then the station called again. *"Jesse, you know we want you. You're our number one choice, but we can't wait any longer. Ratings are coming up and we need a decision. We'll give you until Monday at 11 a.m. Call us and let us know. We can't wait any longer."* It was Friday morning.

I wavered back and forth all weekend. Jilli told me, "This is your call. I don't want to hear about it anymore. You decide."

I made up my mind on Monday morning, and at precisely 10:59:50 a.m., I walked over to the phone cubicle in our kitchen. Just as I was about to pick up the receiver, the phone rang. It was Bob Proctor. I hadn't seen or spoken with him for about six months.

"How ya doin' kid?" he asked in his customary upbeat style.

We quickly exchanged pleasantries, then Bob asked the million-dollar question. "What's goin' on?"

"Oh, you know, we're busy, the kids are great, Jilli and I are busy building this new health business and it's showing signs of promise . . ." I paused.

Bob caught it instantly. "What's really going on, Jess?"

I told him everything—the offer, the money, my thoughts about abandoning my entrepreneurial venture.

"Don't do it," he said firmly. "You won't be happy. You won't like the people you're working for. You may not be able to see it now, but you've set a course that will take you places you've never dreamed of."

How's that for timing? Now, I'm not quite ready to call Bob my guru, and he probably wouldn't like the title anyway, but I had learned to trust his opinion as a friend who truly knows me. His words resonated with my own deeper instincts. But how had he managed to phone me at that precise moment when I hadn't spoken with him for six months?

After Bob and I had talked a bit, I hung up and walked straight down the hallway to my office, closed the door, and called the radio station. I said I had given it a great deal of thought and that I'd have to take a pass. They thanked me for calling and wished me all the best. Then I put my head in my hands and remained motionless for 15 minutes.

If you're laughing, good for you. We've all been there. And I am definitely able to laugh about it now as well, but I honestly couldn't move at the time. My mind knew I had just closed a very big door and a large chapter of my life, and my body was going to take a few minutes to process the reality of it!

But I quickly discovered that I had also opened another door to a larger and wonderful new chapter in my life. Chances are that if I hadn't said no, I'd probably still be spinning records and making silly on-air phone calls for travel promotions. If Bob Proctor hadn't called at that precise second, just as I was literally picking up the phone, who knows what might have happened. But he did call, and I'm inclined to think it wasn't just a coincidence.

This is the first indication of the Law of Attraction at work. Bob Proctor has built his life around it.

For Bob, his learning of the Law began when he was a young man working for the fire department in a suburb of Toronto, Canada.

"I was 26 years old, waiting for 65 to come. I had fallen in line, I was doing what all of the other guys in the fire department were doing, and then someone put the book *Think and Grow Rich* in my hands. That book literally changed the course of my life. At that time I was earning $4,000 a year and I owed $6,000. I had no formal education, I had no business experience, so if I ever thought of changing results, which I probably didn't, I'd say I was stuck. I had no hope. I just figured, you know, this is life and this is the way it is. You struggle from payday to payday. I had a reasonably good job and I would just stay there and make ends meet, but that book changed my life."

After repeatedly reading Napoleon Hill's classic volume, Bob found himself an entrepreneur making an income of $175,000 within just *one* year. Then he topped $1 million in annual income. How? He simply changed his thinking. In this instance, he changed his thinking about money. Hill's book talks about the nature of money in a way that contradicts what many of us might believe about it.

"He said when riches begin to come, they come so fast and furious that you're going to wonder where they've been hiding through all those lean years," recalls Bob. "I read that, and I had difficulty believing it because I had struggled with money all my life. I never had more money than I needed. I was always in debt, I was going backwards. I thought this can't be true."

But Bob also knew that Hill had spent his entire life pulling together the research for *Think and Grow Rich*, studying with hundreds of the world's most successful people of his time. "He had made reference to Edison and Henry Ford and Firestone, and all these real heavyweights in business and industry, so I thought, he's gotta be right. And then I thought, I've got to figure out how that happened. I made up my mind at that point that I was going to start to understand money."

Bob quickly discovered that few people he knew actually understood money. On one level, he observed that we go right through our educational system and come out the other side with absolutely no grasp of how money flows within our economic systems. On a more fundamental level, he saw that we never learn what money represents in terms of the flow of our own spiritual energy. The problem stems largely from a dysfunctional belief that many of us inherit from our parents: Simple blind, hard work will set you up for life. This is a bubble that quickly bursts when you talk with Bob.

"If you just take the time to do a little observation, you're going to understand that's not true because there's a lot of people working really hard and they're behind the eight ball," says Bob. "Hill said if you're one of those people who believe that hard work and honesty alone will bring riches, perish the thought because it's not true.

"He said riches, when they come in huge quantities, if they come in huge quantities, are never the result of hard work. Riches come, if they come at all, in response to definite demands, based upon the application of definite principles, and *not* by chance or luck. You know, Voltaire said we invented these words 'chance' and 'luck' to express the known effects of unknown causes. In *The Secret*, I quote Werner Von Braun. He said that the natural laws of this universe are so precise that we don't have any difficulty building spaceships and sending people to the moon, and we can time the landing by the precision of a fraction of a second. Similarly, when Hill was talking about 'definite demands' and definite principles, he knew what he was talking about."

Definite demands and principles means you consciously identify the things that you want to achieve and the path of actions required to achieve them. It's a *conscious* process of pursuing concrete goals, not simply throwing yourself into a job, working hard, and hoping that it all works out in the end. It's similar to the old saying "Work *smart*, not *hard*." But that still doesn't get at the nub of The Law of Attraction.

Some of the largest companies in the world have hired industrial psychologists to shadow their top managers and sales performers in an effort to understand what they do that makes them so successful. Frequently the psychologists come back and say they can't figure it out. They even express disbelief in finding that these top personnel often continue being successful despite making countless mistakes. How does that work?

According to Bob, it's really quite simple. Most people focus on what they *don't* want, and that's why they get poor results in life. If you focus on what you *do* want, you eventually bring those desires into manifestation despite any missteps and errors along the way. It's not a question of if— only a question of when.

"We focus on what we don't want and we've been programmed to do that," says Bob. "Most people don't want a high percentage of the results they're getting. They don't want the report cards they get, they don't want the bank account they've got, they don't want the car that they have. The average individual is looking at what they *don't* want in life, and as long as you keep focusing on it, you're going to keep getting it."

Our tendency to focus on what we don't want is part of a paradigm that our culture taught us. It's different from thinking positive thoughts about what we *do* want. By dwelling on all of the bad things that can happen to us instead of the good, we divert energy from activities that would otherwise help us attain the things we want.

In addition to learning this from our parents and culture, we have also learned much of this self-defeating paradigm from our formal education system.

"We have been programmed to live from the outside in," says Bob. "As infants, we're told 'listen to this,' 'look at that.' Then we're given a report card, and the report card tells us what kind of a student we are. The report card actually really tells us where our mind was at maybe three weeks ago. It's got absolutely *nothing* to do with who we are."

So how do we go past that handicap? Like spiritual leaders from every discipline, Bob advises us to start by looking inside ourselves. The Law of Attraction involves an important second step, however, and that is to imagine what you *really* want. You need to start to build images in your mind of what you *do* want, and those images will motivate you to move forward each day with appropriate action, even in tiny ways that you might not be aware of, but it's absolutely critical that you stop looking at what you *don't* want.

"Quit trying to get out of debt. Getting out of debt is the *worst* goal you can have. Set up an orderly debt-repayment program and focus on prosperity. See yourself living in abundance. Focus on what you *do* want, and I guarantee it's going to come to you. That's the one point all the great leaders have agreed on: We become what we think about."

To understand what Bob is saying, you have to realize that "trying to get out of debt" is not at all the same thing as "trying to create prosperity." Those are very different attitudes, and they lead to very different outcomes when we take action on them.

One is a negative approach, focused on the debt itself, with a goal of zero-sum equilibrium. The other is an extremely positive approach aimed at surpassing the simple zero-sum mark.

So what are you thinking about? It's a good question. When Bob teaches and leads seminars on stage, he draws a stick man and talks about the conscious and subconscious mind. Using the stick man as a schematic, he describes the top half of the stick man's head as the conscious mind and the bottom half as the subconscious mind. It goes like this: Whatever thoughts you plant in your subconscious will eventually take hold, grow roots, and emerge as your external reality. Not surprisingly, you run into problems when your subconscious harbors negative images about your future. Conversely, you create wealth and well-being when you hold positive thoughts and images.

You may well discover that many of your subconscious thoughts and beliefs run counter to your own good. Inasmuch as your beliefs subsequently affect subtle and sometimes not-so-subtle aspects of your decision making and choices, they have the power to lock you into ineffective and even tragic patterns of behavior in your life. And, as mentioned above, often your beliefs aren't even your own—they are *other* people's paradigms handed down to you from your school or previous family generations. You didn't even shape them!

And here's the danger: As long as we don't examine our own beliefs and paradigms, we keep trundling along, never questioning, never truly thinking, and we are none the wiser. The only hope arises if someone or something enters our life and somehow inspires us to question the paradigm. At that point, it may take hard work to do some serious exploration of our beliefs, including being open-minded enough to honestly examine the evidence that runs contrary to our current paradigm.

This is why Bob says that the first step to engaging the Law of Attraction is to really start thinking, and not to confuse thinking with random mental activity. He remembers a great quote from Dr. Kenneth McFarland, the famous American public speaker and conservative commentator, about the scarcity of active thinking in our culture.

"I remember the late, great Dr. Ken McFarland. He said that 2 percent of people think, 3 percent think they think, and 95 percent would rather die than think.

"I had the very good fortune of working with Earl Nightingale for five years," Bob continues, invoking the name of one of America's best-known early motivational speakers. "Earl used to say if most people said what they were thinking, they would be speechless."

When you hear that statement, do you laugh? After all, everybody thinks, right? Bob sides with Earl Nightingale.

"Begin listening to the conversations going on around you. It's going to become obvious people are not thinking, or they'd never say what they're saying. Stand back and watch their behavior."

When a person starts to truly think and reflect, he or she turns almost immediately to the question of why they're here on earth. This is precisely the time to start thinking seriously about your life purpose. Without a purpose, you have no compass and no direction for your energies, and you spend your life spinning your wheels, just as Bob did when he was a young man.

"You've got to stop and ask yourself—really begin to think—why *are* you here? What do you *love* doing? That's how you're going to discover your purpose. You've got to figure out what it is you love doing, and then dedicate your life to it.

"You have to have a major purpose in your life," says Bob. "I believe there are two important days in your life. One is the day you're born, and the second is the day you decide *why* you were born.

"I honestly believe we're all hardwired to do something. I talked to a man last night who is the chairman of a number of companies, and he said what a person has to do is just focus on making a difference. I think our purpose should align itself with that—with making a difference in other people's lives."

This statement bears a striking similarity to Azim Jamal's emphasis on giving and being a Corporate Sufi. The pattern again emerges where sustainable material abundance is linked to our outward flow of energy and our willingness to give value to others.

"Once you decide on your purpose, then you build a vision. Your purpose is *why* you're living. Your vision is how you're going to execute your purpose. It's a long-range picture of a multiplicity of things you want to accomplish that are all on purpose.

"And then you pick a goal. The goal is taking the first bite out of the vision. It's short term, you focus on it, and you go for it. And the beautiful part is you don't go for it for what you're getting. You go for it for what you're *becoming*. That's the beautiful part about goals, about visions, and about purpose. I believe that is the secret that Hill talked about. He said if you can find the secret in his book, you can have anything you seriously want."

Bob and I once made a recording on goals. I used the example of the New York City Marathon, a race I have run twice. The second time I ran, it turned out to be the hottest day in the history of the New York race. Like many thousands of others that day, I bonked—the trap of too little fuel, too fast, and too hot. It's a really bad combination that contributes to what runners call "hitting the wall," and I can tell you, *I hit the wall*.

My goal of finishing in record time turned into just finishing, and when even that thought proved too much to imagine, it became a series of smaller goals: Just make it to the next water station, then the next one. And that's how I finished the race that day—by focusing on a series of smaller goals. That's what is required in life sometimes, and that's part of the simple secret that Bob is talking about.

Strangely enough, there's a certain amount of urgency to this process of becoming. It's based on another of the most basic and dynamic laws of life: create or disintegrate. Like Werner Von Braun's rocket science, everything in this universe is moving in one direction or another. You simply cannot stay where you are. You have to move forward with a vision and create if you want to prosper.

"You'll hear a lot of people talking about *maintaining* where they're at. They've got their house now, and they've got their car, and they want to stay just where they're at. You cannot stay where you are. You're either growing or you're dying. It's create or disintegrate. If we're going to move in the right direction, we literally have to create. We have to originate a beautiful idea in our mind of something we're going to do, and then begin executing that idea.

"If you don't have a goal, you're definitely not moving in an upward direction. You're getting a little better, a little worse, a little better, a little worse. The tide goes out, the tide comes in. Success means progressively moving ahead, and to do that, you *must* have a goal, something that you're very emotionally hooked into."

Yet, most of us work more or less according to the old paradigm: Get a good education and a good job, then work for a company for 30 years and they'll give you a gold watch.

"You've got to understand that you are programmed to live the way you are living. Your brain is like a bio-computer. Until you change the program, it's not going to change. You've got to learn to change the paradigm. Earning money, being healthy, and being happy is a natural state. If you are not in that natural state, you've got to change the programming and paradigms."

As Bob says, we're stuck in a box. The box is a set of beliefs we obey without examining them. The instructions for getting out are written on the walls outside the box.

Are you attracting into your life the work you want to do, the income you need, and the lifestyle you want? If you aren't, then you might want to take some time to look inside yourself and examine your beliefs about money, work, and lifestyle. Examine your box. Take a true inventory of your beliefs about money, prosperity, yourself, and your secret goals and ambitions for your life. Write them down. Then lean back in your chair, look at them as a whole, and consider what changes you might make to get to your real goals.

Remember, simply working hard at your job is not going to guarantee success. If you want to live a meaningful and rewarding life, you need to have some sense of purpose in what you are doing. You might discover that your current job or lifestyle matches your purpose, but you might also find that it doesn't. Take some time to meditate, walk on the beach, or do whatever you need to reflect on what you truly want in your life. Ultimately, these questions will touch on the fundamental spirit of who you are. When you contact that inner spirit and come to know your real purpose, you will be ready to create an overarching vision for your life and start setting goals.

In our next chapter, we will look more closely at how you can use inner guidance to find your purpose. With Dr. Joan Boysenko, you will learn how to better hear the voice of your own spiritual guidance, so you can then apply yourself to realizing your purpose and talents on earth.

HEARING
YOUR SOUL'S
GUIDANCE

chapter 13

with DR. JOAN
BORYSENKO

Joan Borysenko, Ph.D., is a distinguished
pioneer in integrative medicine and a
world-renowned expert in the mind-
body connection. Extensively trained
as a medical scientist and also licensed
as a psychologist, she is the cofounder
and former director of the mind-body

We must move our planet toward the only
sustainable hope we have: an understanding
and respect among all faiths and spiritual
practices.

clinical programs at the Beth Israel/
Deaconess Medical Center in Boston
and a former instructor in medicine at the
Harvard Medical School. She is a widely
recognized spiritual teacher; author of 12
books on mind-body medicine, including
the *New York Times* best-seller, *Minding*
the Body, Mending the Mind. She is also
the cofounder and program director of the
Claritas Institute for Interspiritual Inquiry.

As we heard from Azim Jamal and Bob Proctor, a profound sense of inner purpose should form the basis of what inspires and guides us in our daily activity with our families, our work, and our community. We understand our purpose by living a vibrant spiritual life that addresses the fundamental questions of who we are in the universe and our connection to the greater intelligence governing the process and activity of our lives. With a healthy spiritual life, we tap into the wisdom and guidance of our souls, and we become better parents, partners, and members of the global community. Taken in this light, the need for our souls' guidance has perhaps never been more acute than now.

Dr. Joan Borysenko is a mystic of the modern age who addresses these themes and the need to reconnect with our internal voice. A celebrated author and speaker renowned for her pioneering work in the field of mind-body health, she is now equally renowned for her work and teaching about our souls' guidance. In the next few pages, you will glimpse some of her insights into the process and practice of hearing your own soul's guidance, and you will learn how to increase your ability to hear and act upon the wisdom of your best self.

As many of the people already profiled in this book have commented, our prevailing materialistic culture seems to encourage a lack of understanding who we are and what our life purpose is. For decades, we have been sold a materialistic "bigger is better" attitude to life, where the focus is clearly outward and not inward. Consequently, we have become largely divorced from the inner world of our own spirits. Each night on television billions of advertising dollars are spent depicting the ideal life: beautiful homes in the suburbs, just the right automobile, a perfect physique, antiaging drugs, pills, lotions, and potions that promise we will maintain a healthy, wealthy, youthful vitality. The relentless message of mass marketing has created a ceaseless consumer frenzy that occupies our waking minds whose activity separates us from the quiet internal voice of our spirit.

Dr. Borysenko began her career in the medical sciences, studying cancer cell biology at Harvard Medical School and later adding credentials as a licensed psychologist. She worked extensively with AIDS patients during the early years of the epidemic in the 1980s, and she was involved for many years with the mind-body clinical research led by Dr. Herbert Benson at Harvard. Because of her work with people at the end stages of their lives, Borysenko developed a profound interest in the spiritual aspects of life and the essential questions of *being*, which so many of her patients began to ask as they approached their last days—the very same questions that our mass consumer culture tends to suppress from our consciousness. Her interest led her to a lifelong practice of meditation, and further study into the emerging field of interspirituality, which forms the basis of her book, *Your Soul's Compass*.

In her work with the dying, Borysenko saw that a series of questions came up repeatedly for terminally ill patients: Who am I really? Am I just this body? What is a life well lived? Is it possible to let go of regrets and resentment? How do we know when we're on track? This experience left an indelible impression. With *Your Soul's Compass*, she and her husband and coauthor, Gordon Dveirin, decided to investigate these questions by speaking with 27 sages from a variety of religious traditions. They spoke to Jewish rabbis, Catholics, Episcopalians, Buddhists, Hindus, and shamans. They asked them what their traditions said about guidance, whether or not there is a larger intelligence we can flow with, and what are the cocreative capacities of human beings. And if there is such a guiding intelligence, how do we cooperate with it? How can we use it to mature as human beings, and bring forth the best potential good in the life situations that confront us? This work has contributed greatly to Borysenko's understanding of interspirituality, a growing movement that is essentially concerned with examining the similarities rather than the differences among global faiths and spiritual practices.

"That's what *Your Soul's Compass* taps into," explains Borysenko. "It's different from interfaith. Interfaith is important because it teaches me about the practices of other religions, and I want to understand those cultures and be enriched by them. But interspirituality is a very special thing."

Interspirituality attempts to identify some of the common practices and elements of soul experience. Clearly, there are common concepts and techniques among different spiritual traditions, and these commonalities imply a universal basis to all of human spiritual experience that provides guidance to our human activity when we take the time and effort to listen to it.

"If you ask a true mystic from any of the world's religions what it is like to feel in alignment with a larger source, how they feel when they're really in the present moment, strangely enough, they all say the same thing. They will talk about that quality of presence where you feel more than your own individual isolated self. You feel connected: empathetically, passionately, and compassionately connected."

There are no exact steps to reach this state of presence, or a precise procedure or recipe for inquiry that guarantees results. You need a willingness to be open and to inquire, and there are a few common practices and habits that many different spiritual faiths and paths use to connect with presence. As we saw with Yossi Ghinsberg, Azim Jamal, and Lynne McTaggart, one of the most common practices is some form of meditation or silent contemplation.

"If you're going to be open to what is and get out of the box of your own thinking, you need to spend some time in stillness. We're just such a busy society. People complain all the time, 'God, I can't hear myself think!' And you don't have time to turn off your thinking.

"But I think we've all had the experience where you take a vacation, you're out in nature, and all those things that were running like squirrels in your mind that you thought were so important suddenly drop away, and your presence is something larger. And often you come back reinspired. The history of creativity is full of such stories."

Connecting with that quiet inner presence opens up possibilities that we wouldn't necessarily consider or discover while we are operating in "squirrel mind." A common trap is the tendency to jump to preconceptions about what we think we *know*, and in doing so we cut ourselves off from a range of possibilities that exist outside the box of our current beliefs and dogmas.

We need to connect with the guidance coming from our soul. Once we connect with it, we then need to practise discernment, or the ability to know which messages are guidance and which are merely our own wishful egoistic thinking clouding our perception. This involves developing a refined ability to tell the difference between your own personal desires and the deeper truth of the situation or decision to be made. Again, there are no seven steps to perfect discernment—there is no simple recipe or cookbook—but some situations can provide a good analogy or example of how it works.

"Let's say you decide to marry this great girl, but you have little niggling doubts. Some of your friends come and say this and that, and you're really struggling with what to believe. It is a huge undertaking to marry someone, and you want to know 'Why do I want to marry her? Is it some of my past history? Am I afraid of being alone? Or [is it because] she's beautiful, and that will make me look good in the eyes of others?' Or is there truly an alignment of love? And what is love?

"One of the ways to do this is to actually take a look at what the fruits of your decision are likely to be. This is a very old guidance practice from every tradition."

The belief of many spiritual traditions is that the fruits of our actions are good indicators of the measure of truth or purity in our guidance. In the above example of whether or not you should marry the wonderful girl (or man), you might simply imagine what the likely outcome of that union will be based on your knowledge of that person's attitudes and habits and your own. Is it the kind of partnership of minds and spirits that will promote mutual understanding and harmony despite differences that might arise? Will it be conducive to raising happy children if you decide to have a family? Will it allow each partner to still grow as individuals despite possible varying interests?

"To be still, to make a provisional decision, to take a look at what the fruits are, and particularly to engage other people—should I marry this person or not? If you get together a group of friends, and say, 'Please ask me a bunch of questions so I can help to clarify. It's not that you're going to tell me what to do, but sit with me so I can inquire,' you've got what another one of our sages calls 'togethering.' You also have a practice that the Quakers have used for a very long time. They call this having a 'clearing committee.'"

The strength of a clearing committee or "togethering" is in the numbers: By having a group address your question instead of a single individual, you greatly reduce the risk of getting a one-sided or heavily biased opinion. Such relatively simple practices can provide immeasurable value in guiding our actions so we live in accordance with larger spiritual values and avoid the individual bias that often clouds our judgment. With all of the messages that continually draw our attention outside ourselves, we otherwise face a difficult task in simply remembering who we *are* and what is true to our inner selves.

"Life is challenging. I think one of the problems I have with some of the self-help genre is that it gives you the idea that if you just do everything right, everything will always be perfect. And the fact is, the only thing perfect is our willingness to keep responding to the challenges that come up in this life."

We have looked at the Law of Attraction, and how we can attract to ourselves the relationships, careers, or possessions we want through thoughts and intentions that activate the law, but we need to also practise some caution in this process. We need to practise *discrimination*. If we indiscriminately try to attract all of our desires, we may overlook important elements or simple considerations of what is truly good and healthy for us, and we may run the risk of shutting out the voice of our higher guidance.

"I really do feel, number one, that the way the universe works is still quite mysterious," says Borysenko. "There's no question that our intention makes a big difference in our life. On the other hand, we don't always get what we intend because I think there's a larger sense to life, and I'll have to tell an anecdote here.

"For at least 10 years when I worked in a hospital setting, I sat at deathbeds frequently. People, when they're dying, will often do this kind of going back and forth. It's like they're in some other realm and then they'll talk to you, and they'll tell you what they saw there. And so many times—dozens of times—people said to me, 'I had this really terrible rough patch in my life, and I see now that it was absolute grace, that that is exactly what I needed.' So I believe the idea that we just set our intention and everything good happens is too simplistic."

This type of "travel" between the physical and spiritual realms is familiar to Joan as she has made similar explorations in her own spiritual life. In her experience, she feels she has seen enough to indicate that the underlying fabric of our lives is more complex than simply "wishing and making it so."

"I'm a scientist, but I'm also a mystic. I've spent my entire life, since I was a small child, with some ability to visit these other realms, and have definitely spent quite a bit of time in a realm that appears to be the life between lives. You meet with a group of souls that somehow you've been in collaboration with, and you realize you've all played parts, and some of the parts are quite villainous.

"In this particular life in which we live, we see but through a darkened glass. There's a lot more going on than meets the eye. And I think all we can do now is to say, 'How do I live my life with compassion? How do I live my life in service to others?' The Dalai Lama always asks this question: How is it that you can be happy?"

Hearing our guidance involves accepting the fact that our intellects are not capable of *knowing* the answers to all situations. I've been as guilty of this as the next person, thinking that my mental gymnastics are capable of constructing a sure pathway to eternal happiness. However, life is infinitely more complex than any blueprint that our minds could conceive, and this is what the mystical teachers tell us. Most will also tell you we are given challenging circumstances in our lives so that we will, in fact, learn to *let go* of our minds and instead trust our spirits.

"The fact is, none of us is going to figure out exactly how it works. What we need to do is simply stay as positive as possible, and that's also what modern cognitive psychology teaches. You can learn to be optimistic, and as the great funny line goes, you might as well be an optimist because why suffer twice? As a pessimist you think about what bad thing could happen, and then it happens, and you've suffered twice! But if you're an optimist and you think of good things that are going to happen, and something bad happens, you only suffer once!"

Guidance often shows up in our lives through synchronicity—apparently "coincidental" events in our daily lives that seem to reflect a major theme or issue that currently occupies us. Joan advises that we always have to ask ourselves, "Well, we've had a meaningful synchronicity. Is it a coincidence, or is it something to pay attention to?"

Synchronicities reinforce our experience that we live in an ordered universe even though we may not understand the fine workings of the machinery. Sufi writer Kabir Helminski has discussed this in his work.

"Kabir Helminski explains how we live in a spiritually meaningful universe to the extent that we actually believe that we live in a spiritually meaningful universe which gives us feedback, which gives us direction on how to reach self-realization, how to ask who am I and what's my purpose, and how do I help; to the extent we really orient ourselves to that, then the universe reveals itself in a different way. We see the meaningful interactions between things, and we see more and more synchronicities. You think of someone; a letter comes in the mail. You need help; somebody offers it. I think this is very important to recognize, and it's very important to stay open to the guidance because there are a lot of things that block our openness to it."

A fine example of how we block our guidance appears in Steve Martin's film, *The Man with Two Brains*. Martin plays a widower considering marriage to a conniving woman who is out to take him for everything. He goes into the hallway of his mansion and, facing a huge portrait of his wife on the wall, he says, "Please! Give me guidance!" and he asks her if he should marry the woman. The hallway fills with thunder, lightning, wind, and rain, and the picture of his wife falls onto the floor. When the storm is over, Steve Martin says words to the effect, "Well, should you have any guidance, please feel free to tell me," and then puts his wife's picture away in the closet.

This is typical of how we interfere with our own guidance. We often harbor egoistic desires and attachments just below our conscious awareness that prevent us from clearly seeing the messages that come to us.

"I think that's the biggest block to guidance. We have attachments to what we want to happen. And oftentimes, if the guidance is not what we wanted, our own attachments and aversions get in the way."

If we can't trust our own desires, then the practical consideration becomes how to listen and pay attention. How can we be sure to hear the message clearly? What is it to be mindful? To be aware? To be open? And is meditation the only way to access our guidance?

It needn't be so narrow or prescriptive. Cultivating silence and reflection is the most important thing. Formal meditation techniques can be good, but not everyone will feel comfortable with that approach. When Joan worked with Dr. Herbert Benson in the mind-body clinic, she says they used yoga, breathing, cognitive therapy, and understanding the emotions to great effect, but at the end of six months, only about 20 percent of people were maintaining their meditation practice in the formal sense.

"I think that it's important to have something that allows you to learn to focus on your inner life. It could be meditation, it could be yoga, it could be qigong, it could be biofeedback and learning to pay attention to the breath and the self-sense in the body."

The deeper sensations within our bodies are very important because much wisdom about guidance is felt physically in the body through sensations such as "gut feelings."

"You make a decision, and there's this tremendous internal sense of peace and relief, this meaningful body experience, which is what self-sense is," says Borysenko. "Or maybe you make a decision, and you feel butterflies in the stomach, like something's not right."

We need to pay attention to the sensations in our bodies. There are many approaches for developing this sensitivity, and not all of them necessarily involve meditating in the formal sense. We can be open to different spiritual viewpoints according to the interspiritual approach that Borysenko promotes, and in the process find the technique or practice that feels best for us.

But be warned: You may encounter serious challenges from some people around you while pursuing this brand of open-mindedness. There are many people who simply don't recognize the virtues of interspirituality or acknowledge the value of some of the age-old wisdom traditions. You might take a lot of flack and even verbal abuse from them. Be prepared to speak selectively about your own practices and faith, and look for support from others of like mind.

You can see the importance of practising this type of discretion when you look at the larger national and international debates on religion. The frequent discord over elements of spiritual faith and practice in the United

States alone highlights the need to reassess our attitudes and prejudices in discussions about religion and faith.

"I think the real question we have to ask ourselves as individuals and as collectives, particularly countries and nation-states, is: What are the guiding principles? It's interesting to look back at the guiding principles of the United States, which said there really is a larger intelligence that we can, if we're quiet, tap into. In fact, a number of the founding fathers, like George Washington and Thomas Jefferson, were very influenced by the Quakers, and they knew there is some kind of intelligence within us that we can tap into, particularly when we sit together to discern where it's going."

"The founding fathers believed that spiritual guidance, in its broadest nondenominational sense, should lead our social and political human affairs. They also knew that the alternative to following higher guidance was to rely on our own collective distortions that often arise from an overemphasis on mind and usurp the wisdom of spirit. You can say you're doing something for one reason, and it's really motivated by fear, by pride, by something less than your best self, and this they knew."

We need to return to an understanding and appreciation for what some call intuition, and others call revelation. Borysenko illustrates by describing how George Washington tried to pass the importance of this mystical approach to the American people when he retired from politics.

"He said to the people, 'I'm retiring at the peak of my power because I have to return the country to you. You have to find within yourselves the guidance that helps make this go forward.'

"This is what we really need now. We see what happened with Enron. I don't think we can trust Haliburton, trust our corporations, trust our politicians. And the question really is: What can we trust? And how do we know the difference between what we ourselves want—our inner pride, our egotism, our wishful thinking, our own limitations—and what may in fact be some kind of flow of a higher good that is possible to tap into?"

To know the difference, we have to engage in a process of ongoing internal inquiry and reflection that changes how we relate to ourselves and other people. We need to become comfortable with a more subtle, less egoistic approach to our social, political, and environmental problems, permitting exploration and promoting humility, and ultimately tapping into the quiet voice of our inner spiritual guidance. We also have to realize that this process of attuning ourselves to our soul's voice is ongoing, and it may in fact take years of practice to attune our receptivity and awareness to the subtle messages that are available to us.

All the while, we have to realize that this guidance and wisdom comes from a process that is universal to all humankind—it doesn't come in simple packages that are culture-specific. It's not just about Jesus, or Islam, or Buddhism, or any other single dogma. Simple dogmatism is driving untold conflict and human suffering in the world, and we can no longer afford to be parochial or insular in our approach. The magnitude of our current global issues simply won't permit it.

This is where interspirituality can play a large and positive role. Rather than pushing our religious doctrines onto others, and failing to realize the changes that have already taken place in the world of faith and religion, we can begin to move together along lines that are common to all faiths. This will require a change in posture for some orthodox religionists in different faiths, but it is essential to our human and spiritual progress.

"That's partly why we wrote *Your Soul's Compass,*" Joan explains. "Old ways of religions talking to each other are not working, and they could easily start the next war. It's really a difficult situation, yet we do believe that there is a way to get beneath dogma, beneath doctrine, and for people to speak as human beings so that we can really relate to each other."

Joan is working on another project to help us relate to one another with greater spiritual understanding. Together with her husband Gordon Dveirin and Janet Quinn, Borysenko started the Claritas Interspiritual Mentor Training Program in 2004 to foster better understanding among peoples of different spiritual traditions. Through 18 months of instruction and practice, candidates learn concepts of interspirituality and how to sit with other people to help them connect with their Source, God, Being, Higher Intelligence, or whatever name feels appropriate to them. Joan and her colleagues hope that graduates will go forward to form the heart of a new kind of global social and spiritual activism, assisting the world's transformation into a place of greater compassion and connectedness to higher guidance.

At a time when things are changing very quickly on our planet, it is too easy to focus on what is wrong, so we need to focus on what is right. The Claritas work strives to play a role in that reorientation. We might not have a moment to lose. If we fail to connect to our higher guidance, and we lose faith in the notion of an ordered universe where love and compassion ultimately prevail over suffering, we run the risk of entering a very dark world. Joan says the research of Dutch futurist Fred Pollack may have provided us with a warning.

"In studying the rise and fall of civilizations, he found that the best indicator of the future of any society was their images of the future. They were self-fulfilling prophecies. Right now, what are our big images of the future? Mushroom clouds? Terrorist attacks? Global warming? What we need to do is to find the points of light, the positive aspects of the future, that allow us not to lose heart. If we lose heart, we lose the game, and that would be a shame."

As individuals, as communities, as nations, and as a planet, we face important questions about who we are and where we're going. Whether we look back to the traditions of Vedanta, or Buddhism, or Sufism, or Christianity, or even the early history of the United States, there is a common theme to how we find the real answers: We are to look for guidance within spirit. We have to do this while respecting and understanding the spiritual practices of our neighbors. Dr. Joan Borysenko is one of the standard bearers in this interspiritual movement, and I'm a supporter who believes the work of people like her is moving our planet toward the only sustainable hope we have: an understanding and respect among all faiths and spiritual practices, and a dedication to finding true spiritual guidance in our human affairs. It starts with us as individuals, and you can be part of it.

Take time to practise regular, quiet reflection in your daily life by whatever technique or method works for you. Connect yourself with your inner guidance, and get into the practice of using it to direct your daily actions and decisions until it becomes intrinsic to everything you do, from buying a car to choosing a marital partner. Here is a message to spur you on your way. Joan says a friend left this on his answering machine, and it helps to state the question in the most essential terms:

> *Hello. This is not an answering machine. This is a questioning machine. Who are you and what do you want? Now before you start giggling, let me remind you that most of us come into this world and leave without ever answering those two simple questions.*
>
> *Who are you? What do you want?*
>
> *(Beep)*

DREAMING

chapter 14

with ROBERT MOSS

Robert Moss is the pioneer of Active Dreaming, an original synthesis of shamanism and modern dream work. Born in Australia, he survived three near-death experiences in childhood and first learned the ways of a traditional dreaming people through his friendship with Aborigines.

"Dreaming is not just about personal psychology, nor is it about random neuronal firing in the brain. It's part of our survival mechanism and part of our evolutionary possibility."

He leads popular seminars and training courses all over the world, including a three-year course for teachers of Active Dreaming and a lively online dream school. His many books on dreaming and shamanism include *Conscious Dreaming, Dreamgates, The Three "Only" Things: Tapping the Power of Dreams, Coincidence, and Imagination,* and *The Secret History of Dreaming.*

Have you ever wondered about the significance of your dreams? Most of the time we may be inclined to think of dreaming as a random activity of our otherwise idle brains, or the chemical by-product of something we ate too close to bedtime, but there are many spiritual traditions that hold dreaming as a far more significant and sacred activity. While not readily understood by most people in the Western world, these traditions hold that our dreams are communications from a hidden world of creation or super-consciousness that is not accessed by our normal awareness. This super-consciousness offers knowledge and insights that our minds can grasp if we are willing to learn how to understand the symbolism and imagery of the messages. To this end, Robert Moss is a dream expert whose methods are aimed at giving us more conscious involvement in our own dream processes. Through a process he calls Active Dreaming, he teaches us how to stimulate our dream processes and better utilize the stories and images of our dreams as important information to guide our activities in waking life.

Robert has taught thousands of people how to tap into the wisdom of their dreams and make use of their guidance. This guidance can involve our work, our relationships, or any aspect of our human experience, but you have to develop a proficiency in dreaming and dream interpretation in order to realize its power in your life. You also have to appreciate that dreaming can happen in waking consciousness as much as during sleep, as there are hypnagogic states of wakeful dreaming consciousness that can be cultivated by practising some simple techniques and exercises.

If you are someone who doubts the power of dreams, consider this story from the many in Robert's collection.

In Kuwait in the fall of 1937, a retired British colonial official named Colonel Harold Dixon had a memorable dream while sleeping in his bungalow one night. In his dream, he is out in the desert when a dust devil whips up a crater in the earth under a strange tree. Looking down at this crater, he sees a mummy laid out on a slab.

Suddenly, the mummy comes to life and transforms into a beautiful woman. Dixon does the normal thing any chivalrous British colonial official would do when he finds a beautiful woman lounging in her bandages in a pit in the desert: He takes her home and washes her up. In return for his troubles, she gives him an ancient coin. This is the simple summary of his dream, and he might have dismissed it as the product of too many gin and tonics the night before, but Colonel Dixon was of a persuasion that took considerable interest in his dreams.

He discussed this dream with his wife and a Bedouin dream interpreter. Very quickly, the Bedouin woman recognized the tree in his dream as an actual sidr tree, and she told him its exact location in the Burqan hills. She explained that the woman he met in the crater in the earth was the spirit of a treasure that he had to go and find.

The notion of a "treasure" had immediate significance for Colonel Dixon. It happened that the Kuwait Oil Company had been looking for oil in Kuwait at this time, so Dixon decided to share his dream with the Sheik of Kuwait and officials of the petroleum company. He suggested that the tree marked the place where oil would be discovered. And the rest, as they say, is history.

"They struck it rich at the exact place he had dreamed about," says Robert. "This is pretty interesting stuff. If you like, we can trace all sorts of fortunes and misfortunes from this event, and it turns on a *dream*."

Though he lives in the United States today, Robert's interest in dreaming began in his native Australia, where a series of near-death experiences during childhood and his friendships with Aborigines introduced him to the Aboriginal teachings of the Dreamtime and the practice of drawing wisdom and guidance from our dream experiences.

"When I was nine years old, I was rushed to hospital in Melbourne, Australia, after complaining of a pain in my lower right abdomen. They found that my appendix was about to burst. The doctors were worried about my ability to survive the operation since I had just barely survived the latest of many bouts of pneumonia."

The doctors advised Robert's mother that he probably wouldn't survive the surgery, so she should prepare herself for the worst. During the operation, Robert says he entered a strange world.

"Under anesthesia on the operating table, I stepped out of my body. I decided I did not care to watch the bloody work with the scalpel, and I flowed through the door and along the corridor to where my mother sat hunched and weeping, my father's strong arm about her shoulders."

If you are familiar with the many published accounts of near-death experiences, this much of Robert's story is fairly standard, though being "standard" doesn't diminish its importance and power. Rather, I believe it reflects the universality—and implicit validity—of such near-death experiences, but what happened next was somewhat outside the bounds of most near-death stories.

"I flowed to a window, to the brightness outside, to the colors of spring and the laughter of young lovers seated at a sidewalk table. I felt the pull of the ocean. I could not see the beach from the hospital window, so I floated through the glass and out onto a ledge where a blackbird squalled at me and shot straight up into the air. I followed the bird and sailed over the rooftops.

"Soaring over the city, I saw a huge moon-round face, its mouth opened wide to form the gateway to Luna Park, a popular amusement park on the water. I swooped down through the moon gate, and plunged into darkness. I tried to reverse direction, but something sucked me downwards. It was like tumbling down a mineshaft, mile after mile beneath the surface of the earth.

"I fell into a different world. It was hard to make out anything clearly in the smoke of a huge fire pit. A giant with skin the color of fine white ash lifted me high above the ground, singing. The people of this world welcomed me. They were tall and elongated and very pale, and did not look like anyone I had seen before. They told me they had dreamed my coming, and they proceeded to raise me as their own.

"For the greater part of my schooling, I was required to dream—to dream alone in an incubation cave, or to dream with others, lying in a cartwheel around the banked ashes of the fire in the council house.

"Years passed. In the highest festival of the year, when the bonfires rose higher than the bird-headed finials of the council house, I was ritually joined to the favorite niece of the shaman-king of this people. As I grew older, my recollection of my life in the surface world faded and flickered out. I became a father and grandfather, a shaman and elder. When my body was played out, the people placed it on a funeral pyre. As the smoke rose from the pyre, I traveled with it."

This marked Robert's journey back to the world of his "present" time as a child in a hospital bed in Australia.

"Spiraling upwards, I was entranced by the beauty of growing things and I plunged into the intoxication of green," continues Robert. "Suddenly, I burst through the earth's crust into a world of hot asphalt and cars and trams, and I found myself shooting back into the tormented body of a nine-year-old boy in a Melbourne hospital bed."

Certainly, this was an experience that was "real" enough to leave an enduring memory for Robert. From this and other experiences during his childhood, Robert knew that there were worlds beyond physical reality. However, as he was growing up in a military family during a conservative era, he found few people in his waking life with whom he could safely share these types of experiences.

"The first person I met who could confirm and validate my experiences was an Aboriginal boy, raised in a tradition that values dreaming and teaches that the dream world is a real world. I met Jacko when I was living with my family in a rough inner suburb of Brisbane. We rode the trams and walked in the bush and told each other our dreams. Jacko confirmed that dreaming is traveling: We routinely get out of our bodies and can travel into the future or into other dimensions, including realms of the ancestors and spiritual guides. Jacko's uncle, a popular artist, got the ideas for his big

paintings—the ones that were not for the tourists—by going
into the Dreamtime."

The Dreamtime is the Aborigines' description of a parallel
reality to our visible world where past, present, and future
coexist. For the Aborigines, the Dreamtime or "the Dreaming"
is more real than our physical world and our concept of
linear time. While those of us who grew up with the material
science of the developed Western world tend to look at our
waking life as objective reality, the Aborigines see things
the opposite way: The dream worlds are the reality, and our
waking experiences are merely a subjective interpretation of
our minds as they attempt to make sense of the illusion of
matter and space-time.

Robert's process of Active Dreaming is his latter-day
synthesis of dream work and shamanic techniques that he
began learning as a child, and his methods are aimed at giving
us more conscious involvement in our own dream processes.
Through Active Dreaming, he teaches us how to stimulate our
dream processes and better utilize the stories, images, and
experiences of our dreams as important information to guide
our activities in waking life.

There are two principal reasons across history why humans
in all cultures have paid attention to their dreams. The first
reason is the belief that dreams have the power to predict
specific future events. The second reason is the belief that
dreams are a communication from a higher power or powers
that provide us with teachings or insights into our lives.

"Number one, dreams show us the future," Robert
explains. "They show us things that can happen, they show
us things that might or might not happen, they coach

us and rehearse us for things that lie ahead. Dreaming is about prediction.

"Number two, dreams put us in touch with sources and intelligences larger than humans, beyond ordinary human understanding. They put us in touch with the departed, they put us in touch with a God we can talk to, and they put us in touch with a wiser self. Those are the two principal reasons why most humans for most of history paid attention to dreams. It's not just about personal psychology, nor is it about random neuronal firing in the brain. It's part of our survival mechanism and part of our evolutionary possibility."

If you're still a skeptic who thinks that listening to your dreams and using them as tools for personal growth sounds like a lot of hooey, consider some of Robert's historical research into dreaming and the work he does with groups on active dreaming. For starters, in addition to the classic "personal psychology" aspects of dream interpretation and the anecdotal accounts of predicting real-life events, there's a vast realm of creativity that has been generated by dreaming as witnessed in the personal fortunes generated by dream-inspired art, music, and film. Just look at the millions made by rock musicians in composing songs about dreams. The Eagle's rock song "Hotel California," for example, is purported to have come to songwriter Don Henley in a dream, and it has been one of the most frequently played songs on the radio for 30 years.

"The song is clearly a dream song," says Robert. "There's case after case of singer-songwriters who've gotten their ideas from their dreams. It's not surprising that Billy Joel would get 'River of Dreams' from a dream."

Paul McCartney's song "Let It Be" is another song that purportedly drew part of its inspiration from a dream involving McCartney's deceased mother Mary—"Mother Mary comes to me." Robert's *The Secret History of Dreaming* features a chapter called "Dreaming Rocks," which goes into these and other similar stories.

Where does this creativity originate? We know from laboratory research that brain-wave activity varies during sleep, and dream states are generally associated with particular brain-wave frequencies. There are also sleep-like hypnagogic states between waking and sleeping during which the consciousness is particularly receptive to dream suggestion, imagery, and ideas. According to Robert, this is the place where some of the best creative ideas are generated or, according to the beliefs of the ancients and shamanic traditions, "received."

"Probably more creative than the sleep dream is the sort of intermediate space in the night—the 'twilight zone.' You're not awake, you're not asleep, you're drifting in between. Ideas rise and fall and something comes to you. I think the real trick for creative people, whether they're songwriters or architects or engineers or scientists or writers, is to learn to hang out in that intermediate state somewhere between sleep and waking—a state of relaxed attention, or attentive relaxation. That's where the good stuff becomes easy."

This relaxed state cannot be generated through meditation practice, however. Meditation and dreaming are essentially different states of awareness and attention. If you confuse the dream state with meditating while seated in a lotus posture on a cushion, you're not entering the mental state where dreams come from. It might work for some people, but generally speaking this is *not* the route to entering the twilight world of dream consciousness, the hypnagogic state of conscious "dreaming."

"This is about entering a flow state. The word 'flow' is a better one to describe the state." He points to the Pueblo Indians of the American Southwest, who represent this state of creativity or flow with a word that translates approximately into English as "wind," "water," or "breath." "The idea is that if you want to get into a creative flow state, you want to flow like wind, like water, like breath. You want to stream with the effortless movement of those natural phenomena."

You can try to make it a practice to put yourself intentionally into that state of consciousness, and it's possible that some elements of meditation and breath work may help you, but you don't want to have to work at it. Chances are that if you are working at it, you will interfere with the natural flow of the dream consciousness, and your experience becomes something other than dreaming.

To dream effectively, you need to relax, so *relaxation* is a more appropriate term and a better indication of how to enter the dreaming state. Sometimes just hanging out in your favorite space and turning off all of the distractions may be enough. You can do this in the early morning when you first wake up, or you can do it in the evening when you are relaxed in bed. You can even do it during the middle of the day if you have the time and quiet space for it. Just don't do it when you're operating heavy machinery, driving in rush-hour traffic, or are otherwise engaged in work or activity that demands your full attention!

You can also use mental games and strategies for stimulating your dreaming faculties. If you want to prepare yourself to "receive" an answer to a question or issue in your life, Robert offers a couple of approaches.

"I play two games quite often. First of all, I set myself intentions of the night. As I approach sleep, I say to myself or actually write down on a piece of paper an intention for the night. It might be very open: I might say, 'Show me what I need to see.' Or it might be quite specific: 'Guide me on this interview next week'; 'I open myself to healing'; 'I'd like guidance for my friend'; 'I'd like to see what the price of gas is going to be in five years' time.' And then I make it my game whenever I wake up in the night to consider what is on my mind. I might remember a dream or I might not. Whether or not I remember a dream, I'm going to pay attention to what is on my mind because sometimes I find I have the solution to something even if I don't remember the dream. So this is the first way—it's solving things in your sleep. You set yourself an intention for guidance or adventure during the night, and when you wake up, you record what you remember. And I repeat: It doesn't have to be the content of the dream. You might just have clarity or focus or inspiration without remembering the dream from which it comes.

"The second game I play even more ardently than the first: I put my question to the world. I play the game of thinking that whatever enters my field of perception in regular life might be like a set of dream symbols or signs of correspondences. One very simple way I play this game is 'What is the vanity plate?' What is the first vanity plate I see in the course of a day on a car in front of me or a car on the street? I look for a message in that. I don't give it much importance, but sometimes it's interesting. A vanity plate I saw the other day said 'Create,' and I thought, well, that's actually great. I love that. What a great start to the day—create. So I play this game of assuming that the world is speaking to us all the time."

This approach is consistent with the Aborigines' concept of dreaming as they talk about the Dreamtime as the "speaking world" and the "speaking land." In their cosmology of the Dreamtime, our experience of the objective material world is informed by invisible forces of creation that operate behind the world of visible matter.

"In my native Australia, Aborigines talk of 'the speaking land.' The understanding is that everything is alive, everything is conscious, and it will speak to us if we pay attention."

The secret to achieving a harmonious life is in listening to the messages that this hidden world communicates to us, and there are different ways of doing that.

"Dreaming is not fundamentally about what happens during sleep. It's about waking up to a deeper reality. We may do that in sleep dreams, but we can also do it in visionary states, or when the world gives us a message in the form of the strange behavior of a bird or animal, a symbolic pop-up such as the vanity plate on the car in front of us on the road, or another case of coincidence that we know in our gut is more than 'only' coincidence".

Here's an Active Dreaming game you can try that is based on this notion of "coincidence": As you go through your day—maybe during your morning commute, or maybe during your lunch break—assume that the first unusual or unexpected thing that comes up in your field of perception will be a message to you from the world.

"Play that game and see what happens. It's usually pretty interesting. You can focus it by turning on the car radio and adding this assumption to the game: The first song or the first words spoken to you on the car radio are your message from the world. Or you can do the 'bibliomancy' game—that's just a fancy word for scanning a book at random. You open any book you like, and the first passage that your eye falls upon is your message for the day."

These are some simple examples of doing dream work by reading dream symbols in the context of everyday life. As you read the symbols, you can choose to reflect further on the ideas and themes that they suggest, and your reflections may lead to more insights into the type of actions and behaviors you may want to adopt as guidance for your daily life.

"We would do better, to vary the metaphor, if we picked up the phone and listened to more of what the world is saying to us. This is becoming a wide-awake, 24-hour-a-day dreamer, looking for signs and correspondences and patterns of connection and resemblances in the world of everyday life around you."

In leading workshops and seminars in Active Dreaming, one of Robert's more recent approaches has been to run seminars over the Internet where he issues guidelines to his seminar participants on some aspect of dreaming each week. The seminar provides an online forum in which participants share accounts of their dreams, their experiences of coincidence, their experiments with dream travel, and the effect of their Active Dream work on their lives. The ultimate goal is to take the information they receive in their dream states—whether sleeping dreams or waking dreams—and use it to guide their actions and decision making in their waking lives.

"The material that is spilling out is just wonderful," says Robert. "The energy and the vividness, and even the poetry and story value of a lot of the dreams and experiences that are being shared are just fabulous. And I notice once again, people are really, really hungry for this, and they're grateful for being given techniques that they can use on an everyday basis."

One of Robert's most important techniques in Active Dreaming is a process he calls Lightning Dreamwork in which people can talk about their dreams in a way that they can feel safe sharing what might be very powerful and intimate experiences.

"The Lightning Dreamwork Game, one of the original processes I have created, is a fun, fresh, and original way to share dreams and other life experiences with a friend or a complete stranger and get some helpful, nonintrusive feedback and suggestions for action. I compare it to lightning because it's quick and it focuses terrific energy. With practice, you can learn to play the game in just 10 minutes, which means you'll have no excuse not to make this part of everyday life."

Robert's students find that playing this game energizes their day, stimulating creative ideas and healing and deepening relationships at home or at work. The technique is simple enough that you can start using it right now, and all you need is one other person willing to play the game with you.

"There are four key steps," explains Robert. "First, the dreamer is encouraged to tell his or her dream story as clearly as possible without background or self-interpretation. In doing this, the dreamer begins to develop the power of a storyteller and that is real power in any society.

"Next, the person guiding the process asks three basic questions. What did you feel immediately after the dream? Then a reality check: What do you recognize from this dream in the rest of your life and could any part of this happen in the future? And finally: What do you want to know?"

At this stage, the participants do the thing closest to "interpreting" the dream, though it is not dream interpretation in the sense that most people might recognize.

"After the questions, the partner says to the dreamer, 'If it were my dream, I would think about such and such.' The 'If it were my dream' or 'If it were my life' protocol is a great way of talking to each other. We can say just about anything as long as we say it nicely, and we are able to offer our feedback without purporting to tell the dreamer the meaning of her dream or her life, which we can't do because the dreamer is the final authority on all of that."

Considering the dream and the ideas it has generated, the participants talk about the actions that the dreamer might take based on the information in the dream.

"We ask the dreamer to come up with an action plan. Dreams require action. We don't want to let the counsel and energy of our dreams stay out there, separate from our embodied lives. If we dream it, we may be able to do it—if we take the appropriate action.

"The action plan could range from buying the red shoes you were wearing in the dream, to doing some research on a funny word or exotic location that showed up, to developing a travel advisory to avoid getting stuck at an airport or involved in a car accident on the road. The right action might be to act on a dream diagnosis you received in order to head off a possible health problem.

"One action I will always ask you to take: See if you can come up with a personal one-liner—what Mark Twain would call a 'snapper'—that encapsulates the message of the dream. 'Wake up and dream' is my all-time personal favorite, and that's what all of this is about."

Acting on your dreams is paramount in Robert's dream work. If you are sincere about accessing the power of the dream world and generating more of the dynamic energy that stems from following your dreams, you need to respond to the "instructions" or indications that your dreams provide by taking real action in the physical world. For example, if you are dreaming of your ideal lover or partner, you should pay attention to the signals that your dreams are providing.

"If you dream of Mr. Right or Ms. Right—you don't leave that hanging loose. You figure out how to get the phone number or get yourself to Costa Rica in February where they might have met you in the dream."

To give you an idea of what the Lightning Dreamwork game can look like, I'll share one of my own dreams with you. When I last spoke with Robert, I asked him if he would be willing to interpret a dream that I had a couple of years ago. His preamble to "interpreting" my dream was as significant to the process as his reading of the dream itself.

"I'll do something better," says Robert. "I will say to you, 'If it were my dream, I would think about such and such,' and I might give you some associations and suggestions. I might, in fact, give you an interpretation—I might give you several *layers* of interpretation—but I would not take your power away by telling you 'This is what your dream means.' I always sort of wiggle and slide around the word 'interpret' because I don't want my approach to be confused with that of the analyst, the all-powerful analyst or guru who tells you what your dreams mean. So, yes, I will interpret your dream, but I will make sure that you do not give me your power, and that you recognize that at the end of the day, you are the sole expert and final authority on what your dream means. I will begin with this protocol: 'If it were *my* dream, I would think about such and such.'"

With that reassurance in hand, I told Robert my dream, one that I call "The Window." This is a dream that I had in the last couple of years, and it was so vivid that it has stayed clear in my memory ever since. In the dream I'm floating in outer space. It's just me, the vast infinity of the universe, and this beautiful window frame, dressed with curtains that are blowing lightly in the breeze. And I "hear" a message in my mind, though no one speaks it: "Go through the window. Take a chance. What have you got to lose?" I feel inspired by the invitation, as well as a kind of nervous excitement, but I also feel a slightly frightening sense that I need to let go of *something* to go through the window.

"What a wonderful invitation," says Robert, and he slips naturally into his Lightning Dreamwork process. "If this were my dream, I'd accept this as a marvelous, fabulous invitation for further explorations of the nature of reality—for stepping outside any walls and boundaries that I have put around my possibility and my reality. I want to travel through that window out there in space. I want to learn to travel consciously back inside this dream, travel through the space and take the risk. I want to see what I can learn, and see what I can observe from the greater perspective—maybe the multidimensional perspective that is awaiting me.

"It reminds me of many dreams of my own. I've had dreams of a frame like that—the frame of a window, the frame of a doorway—sometimes an environment like outer space, usually an outer space that is full of light, not the way we perceive space at night as dark.

"Sometimes I've come to doorways or windows like this in other scenes. I'm thinking now of a doorway—just a door frame—on a Scottish heath, which I associate with Robert Louis Stevenson. I had great adventures when I traveled through that open frame—adventures that seemed to carry me across time and into the imagination of a writer who came out of Scotland, where my father's people came from.

"So I'm excited by the dream, but I don't just want to reduce it to a set of words. I want to learn to travel through that window, and I want to learn how to take the appropriate risks in life to achieve the deeper level of understanding and creativity that I feel is most surely waiting for me."

Robert's comments on my dream definitely resonate with my own intuitive feelings about its "meaning," and this is the value of the "If it were my dream" approach. In my case, I can intuit at least part of what the dream is reflecting about risk taking in my life.

Over the last three years, I have made major decisions regarding my career and business direction, decisions that have involved significant monetary and philosophical risks in terms of how my work reflects who I am and what I value, so my dream of the window feels like a direct reflection of that process happening in my life. It feels like a large signpost that reminds me to focus my awareness on this transformational life process that I've chosen to pursue. It tells me that I need to continue to act with courage and be prepared to take risks to stay true to my own larger life and career goals because there is a "universe" of opportunity waiting for me.

Another of Robert's core techniques is the practice of going "back" into a dream that you've had. This doesn't necessarily involve actually falling asleep and entering the same dream again; it involves applying your imagination while you are in a relaxed state and focusing your attention on the imagery and the narrative of your dream.

"The core technique which I'm referring to is Dream Reentry. You had a dream, and you've been somewhere in your dream. You've been in outer space at that window and heard that voice speaking to you. You can learn to go back there. You can learn to put yourself into a relaxed but focused state so you can travel in your imagination back into that space in the dreaming and go on with the dream and do something more.

"This is a very important process for people to learn, both in order to learn to go through personal doorways into the larger universe and in order to do things like get beyond a fear, something that's challenging you in your dream. Maybe it's time to stop running away. Maybe it's time to go back into the dream consciously, to face whatever is inside it, and achieve healing and resolution. Maybe you need more information. You dreamed of something that seems to be happening in the future, but you'd like to clarify when it is happening, what the circumstances are, and what you need to do about it. You might need to stick your head back inside the dream to get that information."

After reading Robert's writings and speaking with him, I'm certainly paying more attention to my dreams now. I am learning to become more active in the process of dream reentry, taking real actions in my waking life, and seeing how dreaming may reflect deeper spiritual guidance in my life. You can try it too. Here's wishing you good rest, and may your best dreams come true!

LEARNING
TO FORGIVE

chapter 15

with VICTOR CHAN

Victor Chan is a trustee and founding
director of the Dalai Lama Center for
Peace and Education in Vancouver,
Canada. He has known the Dalai Lama
for over 30 years and is coauthor with
His Holiness in the book, *The Wisdom of
Forgiveness: Intimate Conversations and
Journeys with the Dalai Lama.* In 2004,

*In everything you do, remember that
there are fundamental precepts of
charity and peace that inform every
other aspect of your health.*

he helped to convene a symposium on
"How to Balance Educating the Mind with
Educating the Heart," featuring the Dalai
Lama, Archbishop Desmond Tutu, Shirin
Ebadi, Rabbi Zalman Schachter-Shalomi,
and Professor Jo-Ann Archibald.

I n this book, we have heard from some of the brightest minds in human potential and wellness in the world today. We have learned about the latest breakthroughs governing good physical health, received penetrating insights into the benefits and pitfalls of mind, and seen how both of these dimensions of holistic wellness fit within a larger sense of our spiritual abundance, progress, and purpose. In our final chapter, we address perhaps our greatest purpose of living well and being human: How to live compassionately with one another on this planet.

In the past decade, unprecedented numbers of people worldwide have been exposed to the teachings of the Dalai Lama and, through his writings and lectures, been introduced to the ideas of Buddhism. As those familiar with Buddhism will know, it is not a religion that promotes the worship of any god or deity, but is essentially a philosophy that seeks to understand our human condition, with its key tenets being mindfulness, compassion, and forgiveness. At a time in history when global media makes us abundantly aware of the violence and discord in our world, including violence associated specifically with religious conflict, it's not surprising that many people have gravitated toward the brand of acceptance and compassion that Buddhism advocates. From my own experience with Buddhist practice, I believe we can all learn something from its universal principles, regardless of our own particular religious upbringing or theological convictions.

In 2006, I had the pleasure of meeting and becoming friends with Victor Chan, the executive director of the Dalai Lama Center for Peace and Education in Vancouver, Canada, and the first center of its kind in the world. At the time, Victor had just finished writing a book with His Holiness the Dalai Lama, *The Wisdom of Forgiveness*. It has since become an extremely successful and important book, being nominated as the best spiritual book of 2005. Its central discussion of compassion and forgiveness is consistent with the thoughts of many of the people who have appeared in the previous chapters of this book, and I think this reflects how these themes are critical messages for our times.

Since our first meeting, Victor Chan has joined me on *The Good Life* show on several occasions to talk about happiness, compassion, and the wisdom of forgiveness. As an ambassador of the Dalai Lama's teaching in the West, he has shared insights with listeners into why the practice of compassion and forgiveness represents the ultimate path to lasting happiness in your life. In assisting His Holiness in teaching the benefits of the joy that arises from practising compassionate and charitable regard for others, he shows us how these teachings are very much in line with the ideas and research put forth by Dr. Stephen Post and Azim Jamal in our earlier chapters. In short, compassion and forgiveness are part of a habit that the Dalai Lama calls "wise-selfish": You are lifted to far greater heights of happiness and joy when you practise love, generosity, and empathy with all human beings. By being *selfless*, you experience the benefits that perhaps your most *selfish* sense might dream of attaining.

That His Holiness the Dalai Lama chooses to work with Victor in conveying this message is indicative of the degree of faith and trust that His Holiness has in him. His trust is the product of a lengthy relationship that dates back to the early 1970s. In Victor's story of their first meeting, we see the familiar theme of the transformative "conversion experience." In fact, meeting the Dalai Lama gave rise to a complete reorientation of Victor's life.

By his own admission, Victor did not grow up as a spiritualist, Buddhist, or person of especially noble virtue. He was born and raised in capitalist Hong Kong, where he attended school for the first 20 years of his life. The social and spiritual climate of his youth was very much focused in one particular direction: doing business, making money, getting ahead, and putting yourself before everyone around you.

"In the 1950s and 1960s, the mindset of Hong Kong was very different from now. It was very poor at the time, and there was very much the sense of everyone for themselves. In essence, I grew up in a society where doing things for the greater good and volunteering time, energy, or money for a good cause was not a common phenomenon. This environment was something that I reacted against, and when I left Hong Kong to attend college in Canada and the U.S., it really allowed me to get a much wider perspective about life in general.

"After college graduation, I had the luxury to be able to travel to Africa, Europe, and Asia, where I was exposed to a lot of different influences and cultures, and, of course, my meeting with the Dalai Lama was a very pivotal moment."

The circumstances that brought Victor to meet the Dalai Lama were, in fact, "accidental," though in light of what Joan Borysenko said earlier about synchronicity and coincidence, we might wonder how accidental or coincidental that meeting really was.

"I spent quite a bit of time in North Africa and Europe," recounts Victor. "On one of those trips, I bought myself a Volkswagen camper in Amsterdam and drove it across Europe to Afghanistan, which took quite a while and was quite an experience. I stocked up the van with six other people, and we all slept in the van, all seven of us, so you can imagine the coziness of that trip."

Victor spent nine months in Afghanistan, and toward the end of his stay, he and two others, a woman from New York City and a woman from Munich, made an unexpected and frightening trek high into the mountains of the Hindu Kush. This was not the sort of excursion you would seek in a tourism brochure: They were led at rifle point by three Afghan men.

While none of us would hope to be kidnapped on vacation, the silver lining to this story is that Victor's experience ultimately led him to meet the Dalai Lama. Their captors were apparently somewhat amateur, and Victor and his travel mates managed to escape.

"We escaped after three days of captivity, and I started to travel eastwards with this woman from New York City. It happened that she had a letter of introduction to the Dalai Lama through a good friend of hers, so it came to pass in March of 1972 that I met the Dalai Lama for the first time, in his home in India.

"It totally turned my life upside down. I was just a normal Hong Kong Chinese boy minding my own business, and all of a sudden I was thrust into this Tibetan and Dalai Lama orbit, where I started to learn about his teachings and ideas on interdependence, emptiness, and compassion."

Victor was introduced to the basic Buddhist concepts of how all living beings are fundamentally connected through an invisible web of interdependent energy that we might call consciousness. As such, what we do to another we do to ourselves, so it behooves us to be mindful that our actions stem from compassion and love, and not from injurious intent. The relationship of causality between our actions and their effects may not be immediately apparent to us as it can take time for the effects to become evident, but eventually "what goes around comes around."

Victor's first experience with the Dalai Lama became the foundation for the personal relationship that has shaped his life for more than 30 years. While the most visible products of that relationship may be the Dalai Lama Center and the book *The Wisdom of Forgiveness*, the work continues to grow in myriad other ways that demonstrate how compassionate living reshapes our lives as individuals and communities. Just look at how Victor's study and practise of Buddhist precepts is shaping the lives of his children.

In 2007, Victor's teenage daughter created her own small project reflecting one of the Dalai Lama's principal teachings about forgiveness: loving our enemies. That year, she traveled with her father to Northern Ireland and made a short documentary film on the story of a man whom the Dalai Lama calls a "hero" of forgiveness.

"She shot about 30 hours of footage using her video camera, essentially exploring the relationship between the Irish Catholics and the Protestants and the strife that has occupied the two people for such a long time," says Victor. "The crux of her story revolves around a man who now is in his forties,

Richard Moore. When he was 10 years old, he was shot blind by a British soldier with a rubber bullet. And the remarkable thing about Richard Moore, who at 10 years old became blind, was that he almost immediately forgave the British soldier who shot him. Then he went on with his life."

Victor was in Northern Ireland with the Dalai Lama when they first met Richard Moore. His Holiness was deeply moved by Richard's act of forgiveness and his subsequent compassionate work. After being blinded through violence and conflict as a child, Richard had gone on to found Children in Crossfire, an international charitable organization that has grown far beyond the borders of Northern Ireland and now funds education and community-development initiatives around the world for children in zones of conflict. The Dalai Lama was traveling to the city of Derry in July 2007 to participate in the 10th anniversary celebration of Children in Crossfire. During the visit, the Dalai Lama made a public statement of his regard for Richard Moore that Victor says is unprecedented.

"The Dalai Lama proclaimed to the whole world that he considers Richard Moore to be his hero. The Dalai Lama said, 'While I can talk about forgiveness, and tell people about it, Richard Moore is the man who personally experienced a trauma and was actually able to forgive his enemy, so I consider Richard Moore my hero.' I have traveled with the Dalai Lama to five continents and to countless different countries, and I've never heard him refer to another person as 'his hero.' It was a very compelling moment."

The Dalai Lama presided as Richard Moore and the soldier who shot the rubber bullet were reunited on stage, and the three of them embraced before thousands of people. Many people in the audience were in tears.

"The Dalai Lama talks about something called 'wise-selfish,'" says Victor. "All of us aspire to have inner peace, or a high degree of satisfaction in life, and to be in a state of continuous, perpetual happiness. He thinks that the best way to achieve this authentic state of happiness is actually very simple. If you are being kind to other people, if you help other people, if you take care of other people, then the first person to benefit from this act or from this thought, paradoxically, is yourself. You become happier through this process, and scientific studies are corroborating this fact."

If you have read the earlier chapters in this book featuring Dr. Stephen Post and Azim Jamal, then you know the science that Victor is referring to. As Dr. Post in particular describes, brain research has shown that thoughts and acts of compassionate giving create positive brain effects at the neurological and biochemical level.

The Dalai Lama's teachings also echo Lynne McTaggart's research into the physical effects of intentional thought, and the suggestion that we are all connected in a way that is not visible to our common sense of sight. When I asked Victor what was important to the Dalai Lama that he might like to pass on, Victor offered a story from the Dalai Lama that reflected the principle of interconnectedness.

"He was once giving a talk in Ulan Bator in Mongolia. There was a big crowd, probably around 10,000 people or so. And as he was talking to them, he saw the outline of each individual person begin to soften and become indistinct, become amorphous. The outline of each person began merging with the person next to him. And then over time, all of these faint outlines of each person became indistinct, and then it all merged into one whole.

"What he was saying to me is that one of the foundations of spirituality is that we are all *one*—we are not separated. The foundation of spirituality in Buddhism is that we are all interdependent. If you look at a tree, for example, you can see that it's very much a discrete entity, but the tree actually exists in a dynamic web of relationships. It depends on sunlight, it depends on the soil, it depends on water, it depends on the air around it, and this web of relationships is what makes up a thing called 'tree.' The Dalai Lama understands this interdependent nature between people."

Many of us have read or contemplated this notion that we are all interconnected at a deeper physical level, but it's a leap to move from an intellectual understanding of the idea to actually *perceiving* it. As Victor relates, the Dalai Lama also started with simple mental instruction in this and other concepts when he entered Buddhist monastic life as a child, but he has spent enough years in contemplation and meditation to have pierced that veil of perception.

"He constantly sees experiential verification of this spiritual idea—that we are all interdependent, that we are all interconnected to each other, that whatever happens to the other can eventually have an effect on me, on ourselves. So you don't want to have bad things happen to the other because you realize that if bad things happen to the other—to a child in Kabul, for example—eventually it might happen to your own child here in Vancouver, British Columbia.

"And once you understand that, and you understand it not in an intellectual sense, but in a very experiential and spiritual sense in the core of your being, then you cannot visit violence upon another person. You will always have in your own mind that for yourself to be happy, the first thing you want to do is create the conditions so that other persons are happy and well taken care of."

And what are Victor's own reflections on spirit, compassion, and forgiveness? In our last talk, I asked him what thoughts he might like to impart to listeners of *The Good Life*.

"There is a lot of talk about God out there. One of the things that I really like about Buddhism is that it's not exactly a religion. It's more like a science of mind. It's essentially a scientific method for us to reshape our minds, reshape the neurocircuitry of our brains so that there is synchronicity. And this synchronicity comes when we are existing in the moment—when we are in the here and now, when we are paying attention to each individual moment.

"When I first met the Dalai Lama, I went afterwards to Calcutta, and I remember someone gave me a book by Ram Dass called *Be Here Now*. The whole thrust of the book is him going off to India, sitting at the feet of spiritual teachers, and learning that the key concept of life is that it is now, and it is here, and there is no other thing. Past and future are not important. The most important thing for your inner well-being, your inner peace, is to be able to focus on the present moment. If you do that, then something happens to your brain, your neurocircuitry, and your hormones. It makes you feel good.

"It is when you are distracted—when you are bombarded by different influences and different stimuli—that you don't know where to turn. This type of confused mindset causes stress and frustration in our daily lives, while focusing on the here and now is the foundation of your well-being."

The understanding that our brain is capable of releasing pleasure-producing endorphins has been well established through many studies. However, more recent studies involving meditation have shown that you can actually affect the pathways of neural activity in your brain, and alter the brain-wave patterns that you produce.

"For example, a German neuroscientist by the name of Wolf Singer has done a number of studies about the synchrony of the brain circuitry, and how brain waves are focused. He was able to look at the patterns of brain waves in people who meditate as well as people who don't meditate. People who were not meditating showed a kind of tangled web of movements in their brains that were not synchronized or coordinated. When he looked at the brains of people in meditation, or in the brains of monks who have done long hours of meditation, he found that there was a coordination in the movement of the synapses— the flow of energy across the brain was very directed and focused.

"The brain is not disconnected from our body, so when the brain circuitry is aligned in this way, all of our other systems are aligned as well, including our cardiovascular and immune systems, and we experience a kind of boost. The immune system becomes stronger, so not only do we feel better, but physically we are doing better as well."

These findings remind us of what many people have said in our earlier chapters. Meditation alters our brain waves for improved clarity and perception; charitable giving stimulates happiness; and happiness and joy enhances good health, healing, and strong immunity. In Victor Chan's experiences with the Dalai Lama, we see aspects of the work of Dr. Bernie Siegel, Azim Jamal, Dr. Stephen Post, Lynne McTaggart, Dr. Joan Borysenko, and even Sean Foy and Dr. Michael Roizen. There is unquestionably a mind-body-spirit connection that shapes your existence, and you live less completely if you do not engage and nurture yourself in a balanced approach to living that nurtures your body, mind, and spirit as an integrated whole.

Whatever your current state of health, happiness, or being, you can aspire to being healthy, happy, and at peace. We know that some of the greatest teachers, mystics, and saints have spent lifetimes in contemplation and practice of these truths in order to gain their full mastery, and it can be a long path to achieving the wisdom of such simple concepts as "wise-selfish" and the power of forgiveness, but you can be certain that it is attainable. You begin by taking one small step, and by acting on the advice of the many authors and teachers in this book.

In everything you do, remember that there are fundamental precepts of charity and peace that inform every other aspect of your health, whether it is physical, mental, or spiritual. There is a quote from the Dalai Lama that I think captures the essence of where we must start on this path, so I would like to leave you with it: